THE SLIME THAT MEN DO

D1532341

HUMBLE HOWARD
PUBLISHING

Toronto

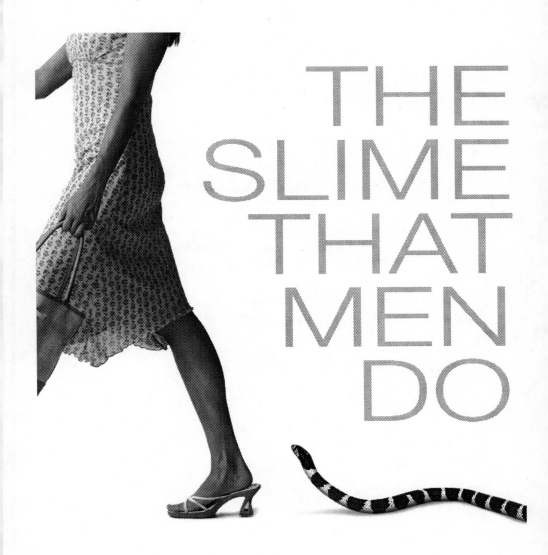

THE SLIME THAT MEN DO

Humble Howard Glassman

Library and Archives Canada Cataloguing in Publication

Glassman, Howard

    The slime that men do / Humble Howard Glassman.

ISBN 0-9782079-0-4

1. Man-woman relationships—Humor.

2. Dating (Social customs)—Humor. I. Title.

HQ801.G53 2006	306.702'07	C2006-905924-1

Cover Design: Sam Tallo, ididthecover@shaw.ca

Text design and layout: Beth Crane, Heidy Lawrance Associates, www.hlacreative.com

10 09 08 07 06 1 2 3 4 5

For my wife Randee and my daughters Charlie and Spencer, hoping my little girls are never Slimed by any guy... of course I also hope they never leave home and if they do, they marry some rich guy who dumps them, but has to pay them a ton of money and then they move back in with us!

....

If you'd like to contact Humble Howard or to book him to speak on the *Slime That Men Do*, go to <u>HumbleHoward.com</u>.

....

TABLE OF CONTENTS

INTRODUCTION

It seems a long time getting to this point, but if you're reading this, the book must be out.

Years ago I did this bit on my morning radio show, asking women to tell their stories of the lousy things men have done, and the response was insane. It seems many women have been slimed by many men and weren't shy about telling me their stories.

I, of course, claim to have never "Slimed" any female but that's just because I've been married to the same wonderful woman for nearly 18 years and before that who the hell can remember!

In October 2005 I was lucky enough to be involved helping the Canadian Breast Cancer Foundation by shaving people's heads for donations... (long story, very nice, very brave people) I thought that reprising The Slime bit on my show would be a great way to have some fun, collect some stories and raise a little awareness and money for the CBCF.

Well the response again was amazing. Hundreds of listeners sent their tales of bad dates, awful boyfriends, husbands who cheated and just slimy guys in general. To them I say thank you very much, your contributions will finally be read by others so that maybe they can avoid the same slime!

To the guys that did the sliming, well hopefully you've moved on from your immature, dastardly ways and are now no longer slimy. Or like me you've just chosen to "forget!"

I also know many of the women that contributed had a personal experience of breast cancer and sent their stories in because of that, and for those in particular I'm very grateful.

So enjoy the tales of slime and my goofy comments in them and if they remind you of any "Slime" you've encountered feel free to contribute to *The Slime That Men Do 2*!

—Humble Howard Glassman
Fall 2006

The stories you are about to read were submitted by listeners who agreed to have their stories published. They have only been altered for clarity and space... **THE COMMENTS THAT LOOK LIKE THIS** are mine and they are only there for fun!

Enjoy
H.H.

ACKNOWLEDGEMENTS

I would like to thank the following people who helped make this project a reality and who encouraged me through out.

Howard Glassman

Just kidding.

Thank to Sarah Cummings, Mix Radio Promotions, Leslie Kaz who worked so hard helping to compile the stories and to correspond with all the authors, Pat Holiday and Karen Steele from the Mix for letting me do the bit and then to keep the stories.

Thanks also to Judy, Bingo, Curtis, Andy and Elliot who were part of the bit and are just the greatest people... I miss working with them every day. Thanks to Tracy Nesdoly who worked on the publicity, Beth Crane from Heidy Lawrance Associates who worked on the design, Sam Tallo for his great cover design work, thanks to Kirby Best and Patti Roberts from Lightning Source for all their help, thanks to Frank Roth for his long time lawyering and thanks to Erin McBride of the Canadian Breast Cancer Foundation.

I would like to thank Jason Crawford. He is the reason you're reading this in a book and not just online. He is my partner (in book — not life!) and has been driving this bus since the day we met. He has guided me through this long process and no matter how many stupid questions I asked he always patiently explained them to me and then he mocked me.

Thanks to my wife Randee. She is just a great, great funny chick and mother and partner (life not book) and sweet and I love her.

Finally thanks to all the many listeners, women and a couple of men, who graciously contributed the stories, I really couldn't have done it without you.

THE BAD BLIND DATE

Just Another Really Slimey, Bad, 1st Date
—Angela Willows

I just couldn't resist sharing this story from "the dating" files…

I knew the date was going to go wrong from the beginning when the hostess at the restaurant held the door open for us and my date snuck in the door in front of me. He insisted that we share an appetizer that he swore was the greatest piece of food he had ever tasted. Given that we had never met, I was a little uncomfortable with this. To make matters worse, he ate directly from the plate with his hands and licked his fingers between bites. *Ewwwwwuuuech.* This wouldn't have terribly disturbing, except that he kept sticking his finger in his nose. *EWWWWWWUUUECH SQUARED.*

I started to think that it was a subconscious action to put his finger in his nose because I had a stray piece of snot on my face. I finally excused myself to the bathroom to see if that was the case. Naturally, I took my purse which contained my cell phone so I could make an emergency call to leave this date.

When I realized that I was clear I started laughing and decided to see this date through. Apparently, it was a habit and not a message to me. *MAYBE HE THOUGHT CHICKS LIKED GUYS WHO PICK THEIR NOSES. OR MAYBE NOT.*

My date tried to order my meal for me but since he had no idea what I had decided upon, it was a little awkward. Even the waiter had a look on his face like, "What are you doing with this dufus?" Through the entire date, he didn't look at me but continued to talk while watching a TV in the bar directly behind me. He didn't ask me one question about myself. I tried to lead him by asking him things that I could tell him something about me. It didn't work. *ANYONE SURPRISED?*

When the bill came I offered to split the meal. He reviewed the cost of the meal and determined that it was more than he wanted to spend and put down $40. I paid the remaining $75. He walked me to my car and when he moved in to give me a kiss, I shot my hand out to shake his so quickly that he looked startled. *AGAIN THIS SURPRISING ANYONE??* When he called again to ask for another date, I let it ring. I'm sure he is still wondering what went wrong and why I didn't return his call. *I'LL BET HE'S WONDERING AND PICKING HIS NOSE AT THE SAME TIME...*   —THE SLIME THAT MEN DO!

#2

Blind Date — Bad Teeth
—Michelle Tasker

The last blind date I will ever succumb to was arranged thanks to the ingenuities of a co-worker. He thought we'd be great... perfect... and was so confident in us being an awesome match that I was sold on the idea. I was so sold that I didn't ask for a picture or too many details. He told me things like he is a total jock, he loves sports and the outdoors, he's a great dad, he is tall and very handsome blah blah blah. *BLAH BLAH CAN BE NICE.*

So we agreed that we would do a foursome thing with my co-worker friend and his wife. The deal was that I was to meet my date in the parking lot across the street from my house and then make the twenty minute drive together to meet the others. I was ecstatic, had great vibes and couldn't wait to meet him.

As I walked across the parking lot I saw this tall sticky guy waving. I felt my stomach bottom out. Oh no that couldn't be him! A voice inside told me to take it in stride, talk to the guy and at least give him a chance. *THAT'S WHAT MY WIFE THOUGHT.* As I got closer the feelings inside me grew worse. He did not look cute, athletic, remotely, healthy or the outdoors type. He had a big grin from ear to ear and all I could zero in on was how bleached white his top teeth were and the bottoms were severely lagging behind in the bleaching process. It looked like a home job to fix years of cigarette and coffee stained teeth. *SOME PEOPLE FIND THAT ATTRACTIVE.*

Okay not the end of the world…don't be so shallow I thought to myself. Just get in the damned car and give the guy a fair chance.

We introduce ourselves and get into his truck. On no, another — "X"… I could smell some serious stale cigarette smoke which was masked by large quantities of air freshener. Gross. That would explain the teeth. From the moment we started driving and for the entire ride he cracked jokes non-stop. Yes I do like a guy with a sense of humor but there are limits buddy… not everything is meant to be turned into a joke. *IT'S NOT??* The twenty minute ride seemed like an eternity. On the way over he decided that we will play a prank on the (unskilled) matchmakers and walk into the house and act like we couldn't stand each other and that it was a total disaster (oh by the way buddy that actually is very, very funny in an ironic sort of way). I tried to talk him out of this bad idea because I knew it was going to make an already bad situation that much more uncomfortable for everyone and would not really be all that funny.

We show up at their house and he plays his dumb joke and I half went along with it but made remarks to let them know this was actually just a big ha-ha joke. We have a drink. I sit back on this perfect summer's night wishing I could be anywhere but here and thinking what a long night it was going to be. We get into his stinky truck to head out to a restaurant and my friend's wife said turn left here (meaning the next street). Well, funny guy decides to take her literally and turn left immediately and goes over the curb right up onto someone's front lawn. *THAT JOKE NEVER WORKS.* Okay you're done buddy. We get there (finally). He looks at the menu and complains about everything on it and questions what this is and what that is. He said he wished they had bologna sandwiches. Nice. Classy and cultured, just my type.

At this point I figure I just want some wine … actually no make that lots of wine.

We eat and his table manners were awful. He treated the waitress like she was beneath him (which is a huge turnoff in itself).

After dinner we go dancing and then finally the night is almost over. I am dreading being in the car alone with him. We drop off the matchmakers and then we are alone. He starts talking deep now. He informs me that he idolizes George Michael and that George Michael is his role model. **THAT HAD TO BE A TURN ON.** He then tells me how much he likes me and could see us totally having a great relationship and how great we are together and how much fun he had. Okay this guy is also real bad at picking up on other people's energies. We get to my house and I tell him I have to get going because I am very tired (of him!). He offers me his number. I take it and make the fastest exit possible. No chance of a "thank you peck" on the cheek. Good riddance. I never heard from him again and hope to never go on another blind date again, either. —THE SLIME THAT MEN DO!

Planes Trains and Slime
—Catherine

I was set up on a blind date with Bart and it was painful. We went to a movie, I can't even remember which one, and then for coffee where the conversation was, well . . . driven, shall we say. All Bart could talk about was transportation. How did you get here? Did you walk or take the bus? How do you usually get around Toronto? How long did it take you to walk here? How long does it take to get to work? Have you traveled on a plane? Bus? Train? It was never-ending. It was a nightmare, he would talk nothing else which was odd because he was an accountant not even in transportation. **YEAH, TOO BAD HE DIDN'T GO ON AND ON ABOUT ACCOUNTING!** Needless to say, I got up, got the bus and ran away from him never to speak to him or of him again. **THE BUS? WHERE'D YOU GET IT? HOW LONG WAS THE RIDE? DO YOU HAVE A PASS? HOW FAST CAN YOU RUN?**
                              —THE SLIME THAT *WEIRD* GUYS DO!

A Change of Heart, Slime Style

I have told this story to my friends and family who have had a good laugh at my expense and thought "how naïve are you."

It all started as a simple ad in the personals (I won't mention which prominent Toronto newspaper this was in). Thinking this guy seemed what I was looking for I answered the ad. This person contacted me and we chatted on the telephone for a couple of weeks. We finally decided to meet and arranged a "dinner date" for the following week. *SEEMS FINE, SO FAR.*

As this person did not drive nor have a car he booked a train ride to the town nearest where I lived. I met him at the train station and we decided to go for a walk and check out what the town had to offer. We chatted and walked for about an hour. I asked if he wanted to go to dinner yet and he said he would like to go back to the train station to see when the last train left. I drove him back to the station and he said he'd be right back (I stayed in the car). Well, I waited for about a half an hour and he didn't return so I went into the station to find him. There was no one in the station and I asked the ticket clerk if there was anyone waiting for a train. The clerk said no the train just left for Toronto. Needless to say I was furious and then embarrassed by what had happened to me. *WHAT A JERK.*

I drove home and called this "person" and left a message on the machine stating what kind of a jerk he obviously was. I never did hear from him and I realize now how lucky I was to not to have anything to do with him. *NO KIDDING…* —THE SLIME THAT MEN DO!

Just Plain Weird and Slimey
—Tracey O'Farrell

Against my better judgment I went on a well-known Canadian dating site at the urging of friends. I ended up e-mailing and talking with this guy we'll call

"Drew." He seemed smart, funny, we could talk forever it seemed. We decided to meet up for a movie and dinner because we were comfortable with each other. I should have known it was going south when he showed up ten minutes late and smelling of moth balls! *THAT'S NOT GOOD.* He had this funky smell! Yuck! *FUNKY MOTH BALLS— BAD.* Anyhow, we went and saw the movie, he bought the tickets and I got the snacks which he ate most of and throughout the movie made this phlegm-cough sound, *NICE.* The sound that makes you wonder if he swallowed a hairball! *MAYBE HE BOUGHT HAIR-BALLS INSTEAD OF M&M'S,* people kept looking at him, and I thought he had a cold, but after about ten minutes I wanted to leave.

It goes from bad to worse. *COME ON, WORSE THAN THE PHLEGM-COUGH SOUND?* At dinner he proceeds to tell me that his ex-wife was a money grabbing pig, who took him to the cleaners and how did I feel about children? What?! I was beside myself! He proceeded to tell me any children I could give him would be greatly appreciated and I would be "generously compensated." *EXCUSE ME?* I kept hearing the music from *Psycho.* But then I thought maybe he was nervous, or just socially challenged so I changed the subject to something normal.

We finished dinner and afterwards he asked if I like dessert because he sure would love some. I, of course thinking he actually meant food looked at the menu and told him I was full. He said he had a different kind of "dessert" in mind. *GET OUT NOW—RUNNNNNNN...* At first I thought this was his attempt to be funny, but he was serious. I was so close to telling this guy where to go! I politely told him I am not the kind of girl to put out on the first date, but thanks anyways. He went on to tell me how he had paid for this pricey dinner, which by the way my entire meal with drinks included came to $23.00 how was it my fault that he ate half the menu? He felt because he paid for dinner, I should at the least give him "some action" *YOU'RE KIDDING?* I kid you not! *WAS THIS GUY FROM 1955?*

Mister Bay Street turned into Mister You Are Singe For A Reason. When I told him that it wasn't going to happen, he started circling what was mine and what was his on the bill! I excused myself to go to the ladies room, and never came back! *WOW!*

The killer in all of this is he called me the next day, to say he had a great time and when could he see me again! I asked him if he was on the same date as I was on the night before!!! *REALLY, IMAGINE MR. BAY WAS STILL TRYING TO GET SOME DESSERT THE NEXT DAY...*

—THE SLIME THAT MEN DO!

Up-Chuck in The Slime Hall of Fame!
—Loryn Menzies

My friend, Sue, set me up on a blind date with a guy I shall refer to as "Chuck" — as in, "upchuck."

I was living at my parents' house in Thornhill at the time, and even before I laid eyes on Chuck, I knew this date was going to be a disaster. *WHY?*

Why? For starters, Chuck rumbled into the driveway behind the wheel of a '75 Gremlin. Now, I don't judge a man by the car he drives. Except this time. That's because Chuck's Gremlin looked like a circus car. *IT WAS FILLED WITH CLOWNS?* It had these giant, rusty mag wheels and this big scoop on the hood that seemed to be made out of aluminum foil. *COOL.* It sounded like a plane getting ready for take-off. I originally thought he had some modified engine or exhaust system, but it turned out he had a broken muffler. In fact, I could barely hear his horn honking (which was his way of saying, "Hello, Loryn, I'm here to pick you up.") *CLASSY!*

Like an idiot, I actually fetched my coat and walked out to the driveway.

Since it was our first date, I wanted to make a good first impression so I was dressed to the nines (high heels, sexy red dress, perfect makeup, new hairdo.) *GROWL...*

I opened the passenger door (since he wasn't going to it for me) and there was Chuck, clad in dirty sneakers, jeans, a ratty black leather jacket and a white cowboy hat with a stain on it. *SEXY.* A pepperoni meat stick was dangling from his mouth. *AW COME ON, YOU'RE CRAP-PING US.*

I was somewhat taken aback, but then again, I thought there was nowhere to go for this date but up. I was wrong. My evening with Chuck was like a Yoko Ono concert: it started out bad and then proceeded to get horrid. *THAT LINE IS JUST NEVER <u>NOT</u> GOING TO BE FUNNY!*

For example, his car reeked to the point that I felt like gagging. I asked him what the scent was, and Chuck said he had been "up north" the previous day and had run over a skunk. The skunk's corpse somehow got sucked up into the engine area and cranking the heater resulted in the scent of skunk essence permeating the car's interior. He said he had tried to get rid of the smell by washing the interior and exterior with tomato juice. I don't know if tomato juice works or not, but when I glanced in the back seat, I noticed several empty V_8 containers. I didn't have the heart to tell the idiot that V_8 is vegetable juice, not tomato juice. Instead, I just held my nose as we drove down the DVP in a car that sounded like a Hercules transport plane and smelling like death warmed over. *WOW.*

Once downtown, Chuck brought me into a really low-rent bar. We found a table and he immediately bolted, saying, "I gotta go to the can. I'll get you a beer on the way back." *OH ROMEO ROMEO...* Offering to buy me a beer was a nice gesture, I suppose, but I would've liked the option of perhaps making my own drink selection—such as a glass of white wine. Oh well. Chuck returned with two bottles of Carlsberg Light (no glasses.) We began to drink and make obligatory small talk when a waitress came to our table. "What can I get you folks to drink?" she said. Chuck answered: "Oh, that's ok, I already picked up a couple of beers from the bar." The waitress then said: "Well, that's all very good, sir, except that we don't stock Carlsberg Light." *NO... YOU'VE GOT TO BE MAKING THIS UP!!!*

I turned crimson red with embarrassment. That cheap bastard had actually smuggled a couple of beers into the bar and opened them up while in the bathroom. Chuck mumbled and stammered something as the waitress looked at us with utter contempt. I was humiliated. I suggested we should leave, and we did.

I should've taken a cab back to Thornhill right then and there, but I still tagged along with this utter loser. We walked down the street to another bar. It was playing loud heavy metal music that I hate, and the noise level totally negated any kind of intelligent conversation. But at least Chuck wasn't smuggling bottles of beer into this place. In fact, I noticed Chuck was drinking quite a lot. Eventually, he was in absolutely no condition to drive. Since it was getting late and I only had one glass of wine, I suggested that we should leave and that Chuck should let me drive. That's when Chuck said—stammered, actually—"Oh, we're not driving anywhere, baby … check this out." With that, he pulled a motel key from his shirt pocket. ***THIS IS JUST THE BEST STORY EVER !!!*** His plan was that we would both shack up at a nearby seedy motel. I was speechless. At this point, I would've preferred solitary confinement in a prison. I eventually said I had to go to the ladies room. Actually, I was making a beeline out the bar to get a cab ride home. Before departing, I looked back at Chuck. He was slumped over in his chair, a trickle of drool meandering down his chin. ***COME TO DADDY.***

My enduring memory of that hellacious night was the cab passing by Chuck's grotesque Gremlin. I swear: my nostrils could still detect the scent of dead skunk as we whisked by. ***THE UNDISPUTED GRAND CHAMPION WORST-FIRST-DATE-EVER IN THE HISTORY OF WHAT SLIME DO!!!!!!! WOW.***

Urban Myth or Slime From…
—Danika White
(WHO CLAIMS THIS IS A TRUE STORY!)

Around five years ago, my husband and I had a very bad experience setting up two 'strangers' on a double blind date. I had a female co-worker who was single and a bit on the wild and crazy side. I would go home and tell stories of her workplace antics to my husband. My husband, Dave, would come home and tell me stories of his day at work as well. There was one man there who he often spoke of, who sounded very similar to my co-worker/friend and we would sometimes mention how they would make a great couple, based on their personalities. The guy was single as well, and so finally we decided to test out our match-making abilities and set these two 'crazy kids' up! When I mentioned it to my friend, she was skeptical at first but then agreed to it, on the condition that my husband and I come along. That day, Dave asked his friend about it and he grudgingly agreed to the date. It was two weeks before Valentine's Day, so we set the date for the 14th, to make it hopefully their best Valentines Day yet! *THIS SOUND FAMILIAR TO ANYBODY??*

Well, the big day came and we were set to meet them for dinner at a nice romantic restaurant, but Dave and I were running a bit late so we called their cells and suggested they meet each other at the bar and wait for us there. We gave a description, based on what they said they would be wearing, and told them we would see them soon. When we showed up, around a half hour late, we saw them looking less than happy at the bar. We greeted them and they were fairly quiet and we could tell something was very wrong. Things went from bad to worse. At the table, he ordered her drink for her, without asking if that's what she wanted. My friend is very independent, and made it obvious that she did NOT appreciate that. The comments seemed to be biting and sarcastic between the two of them. Then, when she went to order fettuccini for dinner, he actually asked her if she thought that was a good idea and suggested she get a salad instead! *WHOA NOT GOOD...*

Well, that was the last straw! She stood up and called him a *prick* in front of the whole restaurant and stormed out. He stood up after her and yelled "And you wonder why you're still single!" Then he stormed out after her. Needless to say, my husband and I were stunned! I quickly got up and went to follow them out, hoping to get the two of them to at least discuss things and leave on a civil note. What I saw when I opened the front doors and stepped outside shocked the hell out of me! I saw them hugging and laughing, almost to the point of tears! I marched up to them and asked what in God's name was going on, and they were barely able to speak enough to tell me! *WAS THIS ONE OF THEM KOOKY PRACTICAL JOKES LIKE ON "PUNKED"?*

It turned out that they already knew each other! They had dated years prior and hadn't spoken since. Apparently things didn't end on a bad note, and they were happy to see each other again. When they arrived at the restaurant/bar before us, they got re-acquainted and decided that it would be funny to play a joke on my husband and I, and so the scheme was hatched. *SCHEMES ARE OFTEN HATCHED...*

I tried to see the humour in it, but it took a while, as I was still mortified by the scene at the table. My poor husband was still inside, and was stuck explaining to the waitress that we wouldn't be dining there that night. He came out a few moments later, and when the re-acquainted ex-flames told him that he had been 'played,' he was furious. He was really embarrassed and felt he had been made a fool of. So, we went home and didn't get to have our nice Valentines dinner. The couple, as I found out the next day went out to a different restaurant and had a great time together. How nice for them... *THE SLIME THAT COUPLES THAT USED TO DATE BUT ARE JUST TRYING TO HAVE A LITTLE FUN WITH SOME PEOPLE THAT TRIED TO SET THEM UP BUT ... AW FORGET IT ...*

A Friend In Slime
—Teri

This is a story about a girlfriend of mine who met a gentleman through a blind date. He turned out to be the man of her dreams. She called me and told me how wonderful he was—he was tall, he was fair, he was intelligent, he was a lawyer, he was just absolutely terrific.

TERRIFIC AND A LAWYER?? Yes, can you believe that? Well, what happened was they started to get kind of serious. He told her how much he loved her but that he had one dilemma, that he had to realize a fantasy of his. *YOUR HONOR HERE COMES THE SLIME...*

Yes, he had a fantasy he wanted to realize. And the whole point of it was that he wanted her to partake in this fantasy this was the way that she could prove to him that she loved him, and prove to him that she was supportive of him. He kept pushing for this and pushing for this. **OH YEAH, THAT'LL BE THE PROOF... LIKE HE'S THE FIRST GUY TO TRY THIS.**

This fantasy involved another woman. My friend refused, and he convinced her that in this way that she was saying she didn't love him, she wasn't supportive, that she was a horrible person. She could never be in another relationship if she couldn't learn to do things like this. **INTERESTING ARGUMENT COUNSELOR.** And he likened it to a sporting event. **A SPORTING EVENT?** Yes, he said "Just think of this as downhill skiing, and all I'm asking you to do is put on the skis." **????????**

—JUST SOME OF THE SLIME THAT LAWYERS DO

#9

Mr. Second Best Slime
—Anon.

A number of years ago I met an amazing woman and her husband through my mother. The woman was my age, smart, successful and not a bombshell but attractive and married to a smart, lovely attractive man. She asked my mother if she could fix me up with one of her best friends, who was the guy she would have married had she not married her husband. Having met the husband I was quite excited for the date. We'll call the guy Joe. **OKAY JOE IT IS.** Joe called me the next week and gave good phone. We had a nice, appropriately short conversation and made plans to meet for drinks. He was going to pick me up. (I thought a sign of a gentleman). It was a Friday night so I wore a simple jacket with the appropriate cleavage-suggesting camisole **THOSE CAN BE NICE,** pants and of course the boots. When he buzzed I came down stairs and there he was tall blond, blue eyed in dirty jeans and t-shirt with a flannel lumberjack shirt wrapped around his waist. **WAY TO DRESS FOR THE OCCASION.**

Ever the optimist I thought "chin up, put a smile on your face and keep an open mind." Well when he looked me up and down and the signs in his eyes were two thumbs down. I started to wonder if optimism was the appropriate attitude. We decide to go for a drink downtown. In the car I asked about his new job as I understood he had just left law to join a company. *OH NOT A LAWYER.* (At this point I should mention that I am a fairly—some would argue *very*— successful business executive). His response? "You wouldn't understand." *OH YEAH HE'S SO COMPLICATED...MAYBE HE COULD FIGURE OUT HOW TO WASH HIS JEANS AND THAT THE LUMBERJACK SHIRT AROUND HIS WAIST WAS STUPID...GO ON.*

Well I was not deterred. I continued to try to find something to engage in conversation that he felt I might understand, but it seems he had decided that the ranking he gave me on the surface he equated with my intellect—not very smart. When we got to the hotel I happen to bump into a friend who ran the lounge and knew that our drinks would be free. Given the way things were going, I was pleased about that. Well it seems we finally found something to talk about, or rather someone to talk *to*, when we sat down. Next to us was a group of girlfriends in from out of town for a stagette weekend. I had ten years on them easy and probably ten pounds as well. *MAYBE THEY'D BE IMPRESSED BY DIRTY JEANS.* After 30-minutes of the "wedding party" I said I was going to the ladies' room. When I got back he was sitting on their couch, so I told him that he should stay I was taking a cab home. I grabbed my cab and learned a valuable lesson—although I'm sure he just wouldn't understand! — THE SLIME THAT MEN DO

Have your own BAD BLIND DATE story?

E-mail your story to **slime@humblehoward.com** and it could be included in our next book, *The Slime That Men Do 2!*

Here, make some notes, it could be therapeutic:

_____

_____

_____

_____

_____

_____

_____

_____

_____

_____

_____

_____

_____

_____

_____

_____

_____

_____

WORST DATE EVER

West Coast Slime
—Twila Allen

I was living in Vancouver several years ago and one night my girlfriends and I were out on the town. We met a group of firemen at one bar, and we ended up partying with them until closing time. We decided to share a cab home and when we pulled up in front of my door, one gentleman asked for my number and I gave it to him. He promptly disappeared off the face of the earth. Them's the breaks, I figured.

About a month later, around 8 PM, there's a knock on my door and sure enough, there is Mr. Wonderful, fresh from a rugby game and covered head-to-toe in mud. *FIREMEN ARE BOLD.*

He apologizes profusely and explains that his father had passed away, he went overseas for the funeral and in the meantime he had lost my number. He was in the neighbourhood for a match, and decided to pop by and make amends. *REALLY.*

Apology accepted, and we made plans to go out that weekend. Then he says, "Do you mind if I use your bathroom before I go?" "Sure," I say. About a minute later I hear MY SHOWER running!! But wait, it gets even better: I'm standing in my hallway, absolutely stunned, when out he strolls in a towel, explaining that he pulled a thigh muscle and he could really use a rubdown. *FIREMEN CAN BE VERY BOLD.*

I'm not kidding! I spent just a wee moment taking in the view (OK, he was gorgeous) and then I told him to get dressed, get out and not to bother coming back.

I'm not sure which grossed me out more: his slimey behaviour, or the thought that this little gig must have WORKED with other women and he thought it would work with me, too. Needless to add, I took every cleaning product I had and scrubbed down my bathroom!

—THE SLIME THAT FIREMEN DO

Anonymous Slime…(You'll see why..)

I had recently been separated after being married a long time and went out on my very first date. It was all very new and exciting to me but at the same time, I was very nervous, as I had not been out on a "date" in more than 14 years.

I went to this "gentleman's" house to have a drink before going out (this man was not someone I had just met, I had known him through work for a number of years so I felt quite comfortable going to his place first). He lived in a bachelor apartment in Toronto, no bedroom, so his queen size bed was in the middle of the one room he did have. In front of his bed were a small loveseat and a TV.

Everything was going fine, I had been there for about an hour when I excused myself to use his bathroom. I was gone for maybe 1.5 to 2 minutes—tops.

When I came out of the bathroom I found my date stripped completely naked, sprawled out on his bed, pleasuring himself. *NICE MOVE, VERY CLASSY.* I don't remember my exact words, but it was something like "Oh dear God." He asked me if I wanted to watch and I said, not particularly. He went on to say how I was the first girl he had met who was not into watching him perform this act. *OH ALL THE GIRLS LOVE THAT ON THE FIRST DATE.*

After he said that, I thought, maybe this is what people do now??!! *NO…OK SOMETIMES IN THE AFTERNOON BEFORE MY NAP…* I have never felt so uncomfortable in my life. I watched the performance and would occasionally say words of support (I didn't know what the hell to do). I would say "oh, nice move," "way to work it," "you sure know what you like." It is not that the man wanted, or needed, my help in any way, shape or form, he apparently just wanted an audience. When I got home I called my girlfriend and said you are not going to believe what people do now on dates. I recounted my story and she assured me that this was not normal and this dude was some sort of sexual deviant that I shouldn't waste my time on.

All I can say is, what a way to re-enter the dating scene. *THAT'S BECAUSE YOUR DATE WAS A FREAK-SHOW NOT TO MENTION...*

THE SLIME THAT MEN DO

Officer, May I See Your License To Slime..
—Liza Stinton

A self-proclaimed 'serial monogamist', I don't enjoy 'dating.' However, I recently found myself absolutely single. I was getting a lot of attention which I politely turned most of the offers down, since no one really sparked my interest and I'm not one to settle.

This guy came in to my work one day, flirted away and eventually asked me out. He was tall, in great shape, big blue eyes, nice smile, dressed well, you get the point. Any other girl would have been in a big mushy puddle on the floor. *I HAVE THE SAME EFFECT ON WOMEN.*

The next day, he came in again, only this time... he was in uniform. I had no idea he was a cop! I know its cliché, but it was such a turn on. Needless to say, I accepted his second offer to take me on a date, and we made plans for later that week.

The day of our date he called just before picking me up to see if he should grab some wine for his house later. I answered with an unequivocal 'no.' He picked me up in his Jeep. At first glance, he was looking good, muscles bulging from his tight t-shirt. I was starting to think this might not be so bad... I was wrong.

I had free movie passes to an AMC theater, so I told him to make a right at the corner. He insisted it was a left. I tried to explain that my friend had won free movie passes for a year and that I knew where every AMC theater was; he went left anyway. On our way to the theater he insisted on making a quick, little stop at the LCBO for that wine.

Having already made it very clear I would not be going back to his house later, I was annoyed (strike 1). As we drive to the theater, we're making a bunch of small talk. He was doing an impression and used the word 'fabulous.' **UH! IMPRESSIONS NOT SO GOOD.**

I commented that 'fabulous' was my favourite adjective. He replied, "I'll have to take your word for it that it is an adjective." I thought he was kidding, then he said, "Don't even bother asking me what a verb is." This was hilarious! There is no bigger turn off for me than stupidity. Judging that I was not impressed by his lack of intelligence, he tried to recover by telling me that if I just gave him the sentence, he could tell me what the verb was. So, I said, "Bobby RAN through the park." He pondered it for a second then reluctantly said, "park" (strike 2). **IN "PARK THE CAR" PARK IS THE VERB.** I couldn't hold the laughter back. I knew then that I just had to have fun with this one.

A few minutes later, we arrived at the theater... the Cineplex Odeon Theater (strike 3). **USUALLY THERE IS A NEW BATTER AFTER THIS.** I gave him the benefit of the doubt, certain that we were not headed to an AMC, and he blew it; he knew it. He had one of those 'I'm such an idiot reactions' and insisted on paying for the movie (duh), since my free passes were now of no use. We went to dinner first—no problems there—then went to our movie.

Just when I thought it couldn't get any worse (or better), on the way home I was asking him questions about being a cop. I wanted to know if he got pulled over does his badge just veto him out. Can you guess where this is going? One block from my house, we get pulled over. He thought it was his buddies playing a joke, but when two women walked out from the patrol car, he started to sweat. He was so embarrassed, but I thought it was a riot! Turns out he knew the girls, and after a few embarrassed waves and smiles, they let us go.

We got to my house, and I'm waiting for it... the kiss. Waiting... "I had a really fun night"... waiting... "We should do this again some time"... waiting... waiting... waiting... I finally perked up and said, "Are you going to kiss me goodnight, or do you want me to kiss you?" Can you believe it? He kissed me—it was fine—didn't really matter at that point. Having to ask a guy to kiss you is pathetic. **EVEN A PATHETIC GUY??** Poor guy.   —THE INEPT SLIME THAT MEN DO

World's Cheapest Slime
—Daniela

I have to admit—when I heard about this contest, I remained confident in my role as the reigning queen of slimey bad dates! *YOUR MAJESTY.*

Ask any of my friends and they will be more than happy to confirm my long list of unworthy suitors throughout the years! I have encountered my fair share. But, here's one of the classics:

Now, I am not a high maintenance girl by any means. I don't expect the biggest house on the block nor do I expect a man to pay for me. I have no problem splitting, pitching in or even picking up the tab. However, if there is one type of man that I will not tolerate, it is a man who is a complete cheapskate! *I'M CHEAP BUT NOT EASY… OKAY, I AM.*

We all know what it's like to save a buck or two, but when it comes to ordering water at a restaurant because you don't want to spend the $1^{50} on a coke, then we've got serious issues. *I'D SAY.*

I should have seen the signs when he would only communicate with me via e-mail. See, he lived in the 416's and I'm a 905-er, so it was destined to be doomed. In our first conversation, he began to get restless after about 15 minutes and then explained how he's paying 10¢ a minute for the call. Am I not worth the 10 cents?? We continued communicating by e-mail of course, because it's free of charge. *WOW*

So, here comes date night. He asks me to meet him someplace half way between our homes and he suggests "dinner" at the local watering hole. And hey, I'm totally okay with that, right? I'm starving to death. He said dinner, so why would I eat before hand?

We sit down, we get menus and his eyes suddenly bug out of his head before he yelps "$6 bucks for garlic bread?? I can make it at home for maybe 2 or 3 bucks max." I don't say much and continue to look at my menu thinking that I have to escape. He then looks at me and says "Do you want to share an entrée?" Um? Okay? Sure. I agree to it even though we're at a roadhouse joint where there is no entrée for more than $12^{22} *WOW AGAIN.*

Our server comes along and he tells her that we'll need two plates because we're sharing. He then chooses the ever so elegant entrée of chicken fingers and fries. The waitress asks "Would you like any garlic bread to start?" leaving him to almost spontaneously combust and shout "No!"

At this point, I'm gagging on my ice tea and know that our server now hates us and I am now considered cheap by association.

The entrée comes and he keeps it in front of him, therefore forcing me to reach across the table for food. I grab one—I repeat, ONE chicken finger, and by the time I finish, he has already devoured all of the fries and there is only one chicken finger left on the plate. He looks at me and says "You don't want this do you?" *OH COME ON YOU'VE GOT TO BE MAKING THIS UP...*

Too annoyed to even bother fighting for what I know is mine, I shake my head and tell him to have it. I should have wasted it by throwing it on the floor just to see him completely lose his head.

Did I mention that I'm still starving? The bill comes and he looks at it as if it had just grown a head. I catch a glance at the 22\underline{^{00}}$ bill and ask if he would like to go halves. Why? I don't know. Maybe to be nice? Or just to hurry up so I could go home already? Reluctantly (I guess to be a nice guy) he says no, it's okay...THEN, after calculating it a hundred times over, he looks at me and says "Well, you had one chicken finger, so a twoonie should about cover it"! *THIS GUY SHOULD BE IN THE THRIFTY HALL OF FAME... UNBELIEVABLE.*

In the end, I gave him the twoonie. Was I about to argue? No. Never! I'm not that lame. It was a horrid date, but it all worked out in the end—we never spoke again and on my way home, I was able to find a 24-hour McDonald's where I ordered my very own chicken fingers and fries :o)   THE SLIME THAT REALLY CHEAP MEN DO

One of Many Slimey Prom Stories
—Rosemary

Here's my slime story… (it's from a while back) **NO PROBLEM.**

When I was in high school, I was invited to my prom by this really cute guy (a friend of a friend) who went to another school. Back in high school, I was a big partier and decided to host an after-prom party at my parents' house.

The prom was going great until my friends, my date and I decided to head back to my parents' place for the party. Well, after lots of drinks, the cute date tried (unsuccessfully) to (how shall I say…) get into my pants. **OKAY, I'VE HEARD THAT HAPPENS.**

Anyway, it didn't work and we all passed out on the sofas and beds. In the morning, I woke up to find that my prom date had slept with one of my best friends and they were going to go out for breakfast together! **COULD BE WORSE THEY COULD HAVE INVITED YOU TO JOIN THEM FOR SOME PRE-BREAKFAST STUFF.** They even invited me to come along! **COULD BE WORSE THEY COULD HAVE INVITED YOU TO JOIN THEM FOR SOME PRE-BREAKFAST STUFF.** Slime!

Your biggest fan (I'll bet you hear that a lot) **NOT NEARLY ENOUGH!**
—The Slime That Men Do

Another Slimey, Cheap, First Date… Yes One of Those.
—Menka Kozovski

I was on a first date with a guy, who seemed like a nice, home-grown European boy at first glance. We had plans to go for drinks, his idea, and we were to meet at the bar, until a last-minute phone call had me chauffeuring the whole night. **SO FAR NO BIGGY.** That's not the worst part. I didn't realize that I had an empty tank of gas, so after picking him up we stopped to fill up. He kindly offered to pump my gas for me … how sweet … I gave him $40 and asked him to put in $30 worth of gas, which is about all my car took at the time. He filled, he paid, he sat back in my car and faced forward. I thanked him and waited a brief moment … where the hell is my change? *DUDE, WHERE'S HER CHANGE.*

Should I ask? *YES.* Noooo. *YES,* he wouldn't steal my money … who would do something like that? *SLIME!!* Ok, maybe he forgot … he'll give it to me eventually. So I continued on the road. We went for drinks, which I didn't enjoy because all I could think about was "is he seriously ripping me off $10?" *YES!* At the end of the night, I dropped him off … and waited … he said nothing … he was about to kiss me goodnight until I confronted him.

"What ever happened to my $10 change from the gas station?" He sat there … like a deer caught in headlights and said "what $10?" I explained how much I gave, how much gas he put in, and how much I was to get in return, just like a Grade 1 math lesson and in the end, all he had to say was "I don't owe you $10." *YES, YES YOU DO.* I lost it, and jus before kicking him out, I demanded my money back. I watched him as he pathetically counted out change … twoonies, loonies, quarters … I guess he needed my $10 to pay for our date! *BUT NOT THE SECOND ONE…*   MORE OF THE SLIME THAT CHEAP MEN DO

Worst Date Ever, Again!
— Meagan Doubtfire

So I was seeing this guy who I thought could have been "The One." Not just someone to keep around but "The One." So he asked me out on a date, just a casual dinner and a movie. He picked me up at my house and the whole way to the theatre he was driving like an idiot trying to show off and it only turned me off.

We get to the theatre and we get up to the counter for our tickets. Here I am standing there, playing with my hair and the cashier and the guy are both staring at me—yup, apparently I'm paying for the date I was asked out on. ***OKAY, WEIRD BUT NOT HEINOUS, YET.*** Okay I don't mind paying and thought to be fair, I'll pay for the movie and he'll pay for dinner. It's Friday night busy we have to wait at least 45 minutes at every restaurant in the area. So we pick one and we're waiting patiently. He's thirsty. So we go to the gas station and he buys a slushie. ***WAS THE GUY 14?*** Everyone can use a good slushie on a hot day but not in the dead of winter on a date. So we jump back in line at the restaurant and he is nearing the end of that damn slushie. We are in a classy low volume environment kind of restaurant and all you can hear is "SLUU-UUURP" from that damn slushie. ***THAT'S NOT CLASSY?***

So finally we get to the table and I knew he was on a tight budget so I ordered a side salad and a drink. He orders the biggest meal (and by biggest I also mean expensive). He asked for crayons. ***OH HE'S UNDER 14.*** I'm at my wits ends with embarrassment. The bill comes and guess who is stuck with that one AGAIN. ***NO WAY!***

So we leave and get back to the theatre and he wants popcorn "Do you have any change or anything?." ***HE WANTS YOU TOP PAY AGAIN??*** So we're in the theatre and he wants to be frisky. Sorry bud, not the time or the place. As the credits start to roll he stands up and YELLS, (not loudly comments but HOLLERS) "THAT SUCKED!!!" So I got up and headed for the parking lot. We drive to my place and in the driveway and he says "Did you know that I've had four girls in the backseat of this car? Do you wanna be number five?" I got out of that car and didn't look back. ***YOU DIDN'T WANT TO BE NUMBER 5 AFTER THAT DREAM NIGHT??***

—The Slime that Cheap-Movie-Yelling-"I've Had
4 Girls in the Backseat of This Car" Men Do

Can Things Possibly Get Any Worse???
—Heather Rose

You are 25-years-old. You are the last single girl among your friends. You have just found out that the man who dumped you because he "didn't want a commitment," is now marrying a 19 year old bleached blonde crack head. You believe that things couldn't possibly get any worse.

You would be wrong.

Here is my story:

Jules was the dorky, buck toothed mail guy who worked down the hall from my department. ***DREAMY.*** He was very friendly, always smiling and seemed to be a genuinely nice guy so when he asked me out to dinner, I decided to forgo his physical short comings and give him a try. ***MY WIFE DID THE SAME THING, BLESS HER.***

As spring had just recently arrived, we chose to eat at an outdoor patio at a trendy restaurant in downtown Toronto. I ordered the house pasta while Jules ordered a glass of white wine and a plate of French fries.

"I consider myself a sensual person." Jules stated out of nowhere as he took his fork and helped himself to my pasta.

"Oh." I replied, unsure of how to respond.

"Yes," he continued. "For example, what do you usually look at when you first meet someone?"

"Their face, I guess," I answered hesitantly.

"Well, *I* look at certain body parts," he said in a boastful voice as if he had told me that he had won the Nobel Prize or something, "For instance, on the subway this morning, I found myself staring at this older woman's crotch." ***WARNING! WARNING! WEIRDO ALERT.***

Having suddenly lost my appetite, I didn't protest as Jules scarfed down the rest of my dinner. After he had finished, he proceeded to take off his shoes and removed his socks, resting his bare feet on the empty chair beside him. ***NO WAY!***

The air suddenly smelled of cheese. ***EWWWWWW***

I excused myself to use the ladies room. In the restroom, I took out my cell phone and frantically called my friend Karen and begged her to call me back in five minutes. I needed to fake an emergency to escape this horrible situation. ***APPARENTLY WOMEN DO THIS ALL THE TIME... WHO KNEW?***

I returned to our table, which wasn't difficult to find as the waft of cheese helped to lead my way. Jules was still airing out his feet, he waved the cheque at me and smiled, "Do you wanna split the bill?"

"Sure," I sighed, relieved that the dinner was over and thinking that perhaps I didn't need my escape plan after all.

"So," Jules said, moving his chair closer to mine and whispering in my ear, "I have a bottle of wine at my place, do you want to come over?"

Just then my cell rang. "YOU BETTER GET HOME NOW!!!" Karen was yelling into the phone, I could tell she was trying hard not to laugh.

"Oh no," I widened my eyes for emphasis and tried to look horror-stricken, "I'll be right there!" I hung up the phone and looked at Jules with what I hoped looked like disappointment.

"I'm so sorry, Jules, an emergency has come up and I've got to get home!"

"You're sure you can't come over for 15 minutes?" Jules asked, not easily deterred.

"I'm so sorry, this is serious!" I said, jumping up and throwing two twenties down on the table, "Keep the change, Jules!"

I ran to the closest subway station and took the train to Karen's house. Sharing a tub of chocolate chip ice cream, I gave her the run-down of my date with Jules and for the first time since hearing about my ex's impending marriage, I actually had a genuine laugh! *I CAN'T BELIEVE YOU DIDN'T FIND THE CREEPY CHEESEY BAREFOOT HOMELY GUY SOMEWHAT APPEALING...*   —THE SLIME THAT MEN DO

#9

The Strange Case of Mistaken Slime
—Stephanie Williams

When I was a teenager, I had this guy call me one night. He told me he was a friend that lived around the corner from me when we were kids. I did remember his name, but had not seen him since we were small. He asked if we could go out sometime. I accepted and we made plans to get together later that week.

When "Cory" picked me up, I was shocked that he did not look familiar to me at all. Being young and a little naive I just figured he had grown up and had changed. *LIKE, INTO A COMPLETELY DIFFERENT PERSON?*

After our date, we stopped by at a local bar. He had me wait in the car while he ran in to tell a friend to meet him somewhere after he dropped me off.

As I waited for him to return, I had strange feeling something was just not right. Call it woman's intuition. I opened his glove box and looked at his registration and ownership for his vehicle….I discovered that "Corey" was really "Morgan." I HAD NO IDEA WHO THE HECK THIS GUY WAS!!!! *CORY CHANGED HIS NAME TO MORGAN?? NO WAIT, IT WASN'T CORY AT ALL … WEIRD.*

He came back to the car just as I was getting out to walk home on my own. He asked what was wrong and I told him I would rather walk, "Morgan." He looked horrified. He began to apologize and tell me he was actually a friend of "Corey's" and that he saw me one day and found out Corey knew me and didn't think I would go out with him so he used "Corey's" name. *OKAY NOW IT'S REALLY WEIRD.*

I don't know why he felt he needed to lie, but I kind of felt sorry for him. I told him that he had no chance in hell dating me now and I would get myself home. *WEIRD, CREEPY AND OF COURSE…*

—THE SLIME THAT GUY'S PRETENDING TO BE CORY DO.

#10

"He Took My Breath Away and My Umbrella"
—Jen Charbonneau

Yes he was a handsome young man. Bright blue eyes, beautiful smile, and great hair. But ladies, don't let charming looks deceive you, because he was as heartless as the tin man from the *Wizard of Oz*.

My first date with this guy (we will call him Leslie) *OKAY* took place at the Toronto zoo. I noticed he was more interested in checking himself out in the reflection of any glass we would pass by. He would rather smile at himself in the windows we passed than look at the baby monkeys playing on their swings. *AWW BABY MONKEYS ARE CUTE.* I thought to myself so he's a little shallow and a little girly. *IS IT GIRLY TO THINK BABY MONKEYS ARE CUTE? OOPS.*

The day went on and the clouds went from white to grey. I felt a drop. Then suddenly it poured. Good thing I had my umbrella with me. I opened the umbrella, raised it over my head. Leslie says "hey babe can you hook me up with that, I don't want to ruin my hair." *COME ON, HE DID NOT SAY "BABE!"*

I look at him in a puzzled way, handed it over and by the time it finished raining I looked like a wet dog. *AWWW WET DOGS ARE CUTE TOO.* He really did take my breath away when we first met but he also took my umbrella, what a jerk!

—The Slime That Conceited Asses Do.

More Bad, Slimey-Dates
—Catherine Wood

My story of a date gone VERY wrong was in February several years ago, when I was too young to know better. I should have known that this was not going to be good when I had to pick him up. Always a bad sign. When I picked him up, he asked if we could just make a quick stop before we went out *ALSO A BAD SIGN, NOW YOU'RE NOT ON A DATE, YOU'RE RUNNING ERRANDS!*

I didn't have a problem with that so I followed his directions and we ended up at a basement apartment in Scarborough. He asked me to come in with him, so I did (told you, young and stupid).

As I walked through the door, I noticed a baby car seat on the floor, at that point I questioned him further about way we were here. He told me that he just moved out of this apartment and just wanted to pick up a few things. As I was standing and waiting for him, a woman walked in. Apparently, this was his recently ex-girlfriend, with whom he had a baby. *NOT EXACTLY A DREAM-DATE SCENARIO.* Well, they started yelling at each other while I tried to blend into the background. After a minute of this, I turned to leave, and he followed me. So we got into my car and he now wanted to proceed with the date. *WELL OF COURSE HE DID, AFTER ALL THINGS WE'RE GOING SO WELL ALREADY.*

He directed me to where he now wanted to go, which turned out to be a coffee shop. We stayed for a couple of hours of awkward talking, since this was a first date and I did not want to talk about his ex. I finally made the excuse that I had to get up early in the morning, so I needed to take him home. It was now reasonably late, and it had been snowing, so the roads were covered in snow. Now, to give you a little bit of a description, he was at least 6'4" and a bouncer in a bar, so he was a very big man. I, on the other hand am 5'2" and very petite. I was wearing a skirt and high, spiked heels. Hey, it was the '80s. *SURE, WE ALL WORE THAT OUTFIT THEN.*

Well, on the way home, my car broke down, and of course it was in the middle of nowhere. We were north of the city, but I knew that there was a gas station not far and it was all down hill. So, I politely asked if he would push the car. He replied. "No way, I'm not pushing! It's your car, you push!" So, I stopped being nice, and told him to get out! *WOW, I'M SURPRISED THINGS DIDN'T WORK OUT, THANKS TO…*

—THE SLIME THAT MEN DO

Wedding Bell Slime
—Traci Tomkin

I think I have a good slime story.

I went on a date to a wedding many years ago. If that sounds very romantic, well, think again. I had been introduced to this man through my boss, and he was one of those dreamy Swedes: good looks, tall, blond, blue eyes, the whole package. *WAS HIS NAME? MATTS?* We seemed to be having a good time (at least that's what I thought). The wedding was a little unusual, granted, but nevertheless, a wedding. It was held in a barn way out in the country, sort of like the old country weddings, where the preacher performs the ceremony and then the whole town celebrates. *SOUNDS FUN, LIKE AN EPISODE OF "LITTLE*

HOUSE ON THE PRAIRIE." Well that's what this one was like. To make the wedding more special to me, it was my cousin who was getting married. *COUSINS ARE NICE.*

We were assigned our tables, my date ordered some drinks, and we watched the proceedings. I noticed that there was a little more than ordering when he ordered the second round of drinks from the waitress. *A LITTLE SOMETHING GOING ON?*

About half an hour into the meal part of the wedding, my date disappeared—supposedly to go to the washroom and then to get his jacket out of the car. Well he was gone longer than the time it took to do those two things. Thinking that he may have fallen into the outhouse, I went to look for him. *OUTHOUSES ARE A GOOD PLACE FOR SLIME.*

Well, I finally found him—and the waitress—in the back of the barn, behind the hay, doing the nasty! *YOU NEVER SAW THAT ON "LITTLE HOUSE"!*

He didn't know that I had seen this, so I quietly went back to the table, waited till he returned, promptly told him to take me home (unfortunately for me it was about an hour's drive, otherwise, I would have gotten home some other way). *WASN'T HE ALL COVERED IN STRAW!* Needless to say I never saw or spoke to him again.

—THE SLIME THAT DREAMY (HORNY) SWEDISH MEN DO!

No Wallet, No Money But Plenty Of Slime!
—Crystal Moore

Wait until you hear this one.

I had been dating this guy for only about three weeks when I had decided I wanted to double date with my sister and her husband. *THESE THINGS ALWAYS START OUT SOUNDING SO INNOCENT.*

We decided to just go to a local restaurant/bar. Everything was going great until close to the end of the dinner when my date tells me that he has no money with him and he doesn't have his wallet. At first this just threw me off—Who comes out without their wallet? I had just $5.00 in my wallet because I'd lost my debit card a couple days earlier. Did I mention that my date told me to tell my sister and brother-in-law that he was treating because he wanted to make a good impression. *THESE THINGS HAPPEN.*

Then my brother-in-law said he needed some air and my sister went with him. So I decided that this was a good time to ask them to spot us the money. So, of course, they said that it was not a problem but made it a point to say that my pal was weird to not bring money, but they were okay with it. *YEAH BUT SO FAR IT'S NOT SO SO WEIRD.*

So when they came back Big Boy says okay lets go. And we all turn to him like "don't we have to pay," he says no he forgot that he had money in his pocket. Which again made no sense because the bill was $140.00. *AH HA, NOW COMES THE SKETCHY PARTS...*

A couple days later I was talking with my sister and she tells me my brother-in-law is missing $180.00 from his wallet—and that he always leaves his wallet in the side pocket of his jacket! That's when it all came together; this guy stole from my brother-in-law to pay for the meal. I called him and confronted him on his answering machine because he did not answer. Let's just say that he never called me back and every time I called I got his machine. Moral of the story do not let anyone meet your family without doing a through background check. *OKAY, THE SLIME THAT EMBARRASSED GUYS WHO FORGOT THEIR WALLETS BUT STOLE MONEY FROM SOME OTHER DUDE AND THEN DENY IT DO.*

Hey That Slime Is Stealing...
—Submitted by S.K.N.

Once upon a time there was an innocent girl—me. I'd just started my first full time office job when the warehouse foreman came to tell me there was a young man who wished to become acquainted with me. I agreed to meet him outside the company doors at quitting time. He was blonde, blue-eyed and drove a sporty Camaro. *COOL.* Superficially

I was already impressed. When he asked me out as he was driving me home, I was doubly impressed. *SO FAR NO SLIME, BUT WE ALL KNOW IT'S COMING...*

A couple of nights later, we went to a restaurant and the first thing he asked me was how large of a purse I was carrying. *MAKES ONE WONDER...* Made me wonder. Throughout dinner, we talked and then afterwards in the car, he began handing me the salt and pepper shakers from the table, assorted cutlery, a glass etc. *OH COME ON...* He was dazed and confused at my horror and outrage.

Needless to say I was far from impressed by his stealing and there were NO further dates. *NO? I WONDER WHY...* Too bad he didn't know how to steal a heart rather than a bunch of tableware.

—THE SLIME THAT KLEPTOMANIACS DO

Call Display? Why Look, It's Slime on the Phone!
—Carrie Whiteduck

Hey Howard,

A college friend of mine had been single for the past two years. He did speed dating, internet dating and only god knows where else. *OKAY.*

I went out for dinner with him a couple of weeks ago and he told me of an embarrassing situation. After he goes on a date with someone he determines whether or not he would like to see them again, which what we all do, not a big deal. However, if he doesn't wish to see them again he renames them on his cell phone as a don't answer, instead of letting them know that he is not interested. *WELL THAT'S SORT OF SLIMEY.*

So one day one of the "don't answers" called him from another phone and asked him if he would like to go out for dinner. He didn't really want to but he said yes. *MAYBE HE WAS HUNGRY.* During dinner he was surprised that he was having a good time. They had decided that they were going to go back to her house to watch movies. She asked if she could use his cell phone to call her roommate to let her know that they were coming back, and he said sure without even thinking. *UH OH.*

When she dialed her number she saw don't answer appear, the smile from her face dropped and she looked at him as said very loud and in annoyed voice what the hell is this? He just looked at her like a deer caught in the headlights of a car, and said nothing. She told him if he didn't want to see her again he could have just said so. *YEAH.* He then watched her grab her purse and walk out the door in the middle of dinner with everyone looking at him. He was humiliated, but said that since then a couple more of them have made the "don't answer list".

It doesn't sound like he's learned his lesson. I told him to stop being a wimp (though I used a different word—) *DID IT RHYME WITH "STICK" OR "TUSSY"?* and give women the common courtesy of letting them know if he is not interested.

—THE SLIME THAT MEN DO

#16

Cheap, Slimey, Momma's Boy
—Manon Grey

When living in Montreal, my sister and I would go dancing every Friday and Saturday night. One night I met this guy there—he was very tall, and very good looking. We had a couple of dates and it didn't take long for me to notice that not only was he the cheapest "b" I ever met, but all he talked about was himself, his car and his "mother." *CHEAP "B" EH? HMMM WHAT COULD THAT BE... DOES IT RHYME WITH "RASTURD"? ANYWAY.*

On mother's day weekend, he asked me to go with him and see his "mother." I agreed and recommended that we stopped somewhere to buy her flowers. He argued the point for a while saying that all his mother wants is his presence and a kiss. That she doesn't want or need anything else. *WOW.* Not having a mother myself since the age of 10, I argued it right back and told him that showing appreciation for his mother could involve more than just his good looks. So we stopped at a "dépaneur" (convenience store). *I LOVE THOSE, YOU CAN BUY BEER AND WINE IN THEM.* We looked at the pretty bouquets they were selling, ranging anywhere from $5 to $10. His final choice was a single red rose that looked about three weeks old and was on special at 99¢. I couldn't believe that's what he chose, claiming that his mother would find it very touching that her son brought her a single red rose. *OH YEAH, SO TOUCHING.* I wanted to throw up. I was thinking, if that's how he shows appreciation to his own mother, I can already imagine what his future wife will have to go through. So we get to his mother's at lunch time. She's all excited to see her "baby." Yes, I found a Mama's boy that can do no wrong. Not only did I have to listen to him talk about himself all the time, I had to hear it all over again by "mother." Right after lunch, he told us he was leaving to see someone and would be back in a couple of minutes. He insisted that I stay and keep his mother company. I wasn't impressed but I didn't want to disappoint "mother" so I stayed behind. The guy left at 1 PM and didn't come back until after 6 PM. *NO WAY.* He left me for the entire afternoon with "mother." When he came back, I was not too impressed and asked him where he'd been. Wouldn't you know it: the guy was a golfer and decided to go spend the afternoon at the driving range... *NO WAY— SQUARED.*

I told him not to bother asking me out again...

—THE SLIME THAT CHEAP, MAMMA'S BOY–GOLFERS DO

Have your own WORST DATE EVER story?

E-mail your story to **slime@humblehoward.com** and it could be included in our next book, *The Slime That Men Do 2!*

Here, make some notes, it could be therapeutic:

_____

_____

_____

_____

_____

_____

_____

_____

_____

_____

_____

_____

_____

_____

_____

THE SLIME FROM ONLINE

Slime on the Internet?? Who Knew!
—Mindy Wyatt

Well in today's age of internet dating, a lot of trust has to be given when meeting someone from online. If you start dating this person you have to trust that they are not still "trolling" on the site for others. *OK SO FAR.*

I met a LOSER and dated him for six months. Then we were joking around on his computer one day and I noticed all of his passwords were written right beside his computer. I asked how often he checks the profile he used when he met me. He said that he rarely checked it. I laughed and said that we should check it for fun and he got REALLY uneasy. *NOW HE'S THINKING MAYBE THERE WAS A BETTER PLACE TO LEAVE HIS PASSWORDS THAN RIGHT NEXT TO HIS COMPUTER.*

I knew that he had been using the account by the way he was acting. I got my way and we looked at the account. In his sent folder were crude and sexual comments written to other women. One girl wanted to help him relieve frustration in a way that only a wife or girlfriend should assist, he responded by telling her that he wanted her to help him, too!

Needless to say, our relationship ended that day. Apparently he enjoyed living in the fantasy world he created online more than dedicating himself to an honest relationship with me.

Karma is wonderful as he is jobless now and can't even afford the internet!! HA HA! Guess he won't be finding a new girlfriend that way anytime soon! *AT LEAST SOMEONE NEW WON'T HAVE TO PUT UP WITH...* —THE SLIME THAT MEN DO.

Internet Idiot
—MJ

A few years ago I was in a dating slump and having difficulty meeting nice, single men. A friend coerced me into joining Lavalife. Truthfully I was a little hesitant. After all, I had heard so many scary Internet stories. But what the heck, I joined.

It didn't take long for me to meet someone. Some e-mails and telephone chatting later we decided to meet. And after a few dates and several phone calls later he invited me to his place for the weekend. We had a great time (without having sex) **THAT CAN HAPPEN,** and I really started to think this guy was a true gem. **WRONG.** A one-of-a-kind guy. After the weekend was over we had agreed to chat during the week and make some plans for the following week. He would call me or I would call him. No big deal.

By Wednesday I hadn't heard anything I started thinking I had been given the "I'll call ya" line. *I GET THAT ALL THE TIME—FROM MY WIFE*

I was hesitant but I decided to find out for sure so I called and left a nice message asking about the weekend plans. By Friday night I still hadn't heard anything so I decided to call one more time and then forget him. I dialed the number and the lovely Bell Canada Lady came on the line and said "I'm sorry the party you are trying to reach does not wish to speak with you at this time. You have been Call Blocked." WHAT THE? *"WHAT THE?"*

I've been dumped before, even on the phone but NEVER via the phone company. I was blown away. I was angry. I sent him a nasty e-mail that made me feel good about myself. *GOOD*

Weeks went by and I forgot all about him. But one morning I check my e-mail and sure enough I had one from this Slime with the subject SORRY. He went on and on about how sorry he was and how much he really liked me and thought he deserved a second chance. I wrote him back saying Thanks but NO THANKS. And then I immediately deleted my Lavalife file and have officially given up meeting men on the Internet. *ON THE INTERNET OR IN PERSON...*

—THE SLIME THAT MEN DO

Not So Slimey As Weird
—Becky Benson

The STRANGEST date I've ever been on was a couple of weeks ago.

I met the guy online and we had spoken on the phone a number of times. When we finally decided to meet up and go out, the weather was terrible, he kept me waiting for nearly 20 minutes as he finished getting ready, five minutes after he was in the car we got into a car accident. My car had to be towed and it took a while to get a courtesy car. *HOW DO YOU GET A COURTESY CAR??* Then it was off to the restaurant where two children who were not being supervised by their parents proceeded to hit us with their chop sticks. We didn't think it could get any worse but at the end of the evening when we headed back to the car there was an intoxicated man urinating on my courtesy car. Have you EVER heard of a more awkward date?!! *YES AS A MATTER OF FACT I HAVE, JUST FLIP A PAGE OR TWO...THE SLIME THAT INTOXICATED GUYS DO ON UH COURTESY CARS.*

Internet Guys Can Be A Bit Slimey and Cheap
—Robin

So, I met this guy online who is listed as 'self employed.' *UH OH* We corresponded for a while and talked on the phone and finally decided to meet at a local restaurant-bar.

I got there first and went to the bar and ordered a drink. Forty minutes later he showed up with an excuse that he got lost. *NICE START.*

We started to chat and I realized that he is not really 'self employed' but more like 'unemployed' and begrudged me for my job and my success. We had ordered some food and drinks, and then he excused himself to go to the washroom. While he was gone, I decided to check my voicemail on my phone after noticing that someone had called. He returned from the washroom and scolded me for checking my voice-mail when on a date **PEOPLE WHO ARE LATE SHOULDN'T SCOLD.** I then excused myself to go to the washroom; when I returned, he was gone leaving me with a $35 bar and food bill. **KIND OF A DATE-AND-DASH.**

The bartender and I had a good laugh about this awful date and I never called him or wrote to him to tell him what a loser he was. **MAYBE YOU SHOULD HAVE GONE OUT WITH THE BARTENDER, AT LEAST HE WOULD HAVE BEEN ABLE TO FIND THE PLACE...**

—THE SLIME THAT MEN DO

Internet Slime Strikes Again
—Anon.

A few years back I met a man through an online service. There was instant chemistry between us. He was attractive, funny, athletic, ambitious, and attentive. We began dating and things were going very well. He had is own business (or so I thought). He said all the right things and I was falling. He came into my life a couple of years after I had separated from another man and I felt I was ready to let someone in again.

We dated for about four or five months. Over time, some things started to happen that sent up a flag here and there for me, things to do with money, work, and addresses of residence. But when I confronted him he had all the right answers and quelled my concerns. Unbeknownst to me, he went through my things and got my bank account number and began depositing cheques into my account and withdrawing money immediately after. **THAT'S NOT GOOD.** This all happened within a period of about one week. Needless to say they all bounced—to the tune of about $4,000. My bank called me and said that they were freezing my accounts as I was in overdraft for $4,000 and that I had to come in and sign a promissory note to repay the money within a certain time period before they took legal action, and even though they knew this was not my doing, it was my account. *WHAT HAPPENED TO ATTRACTIVE, FUNNY, ATHLETIC BLAH BLAH BLAH?* He also managed to get three $500 withdrawals from my credit card. I told him that if the money was not back in my account within 24 hours I was calling the police, which I was going to do anyway but thought I might at least get my account straightened out first.

CAN IT GET WORSE?? LIKE, OH I DON'T KNOW, TRY AND BORROW SOME MONEY FROM YOUR 80-YEAR-OLD MOM!

He was in a panic needless to say and was running around sleepless for the next couple of days trying to get money from people. But then I get a call from my 80-year-old mother who says that he was just at her house and told her that I said it was alright if he asked to borrow $2,000 from her! So of course being the sweetheart that she is and the sweet talker that he was she wrote him a cheque, but he had her put it in the name of someone else as he wasn't going to be able to cash it of course. I freaked but was unable to get in contact with him. I sent him e-mails letting him know that he had just done the unspeakable and I was not going to let him get away with it.

He tried to back-peddle and made up excuses and of course but would not call me or meet me anywhere, he only sent e-mails. I saved them all and handed them over to the police later. *WOW. THIS GUY IS LIKE A MOVIE CROOK.*

I started making some calls only to discover that the business he told me about was not his (although he had business cards in that name), then the address he was staying at was not really his. I found another card with an address on it after digging through boxes of his things. I drove to that address that night with a g/f in tow...*G/F? GIRLFRIEND?* It was not in the nicest part of T.O. I rang the buzzer and low and behold he answered, caught totally off guard, but when he heard my voice he hung up. I rang and rang again until someone else answered and said that he wasn't there.

The next day I had a friend do some digging for me and found out that he was on parole. I managed to get his parole officer's name and made a call. I told her what had happened and asked what he had been in jail for and the officer was not able to actually come right out and tell me but I still got the answer I needed—FRAUD!!!! *SURPRISE...* Numerous other women were caught in the same scenario as mine. At the time he was with me, he was actually working for a promotions company and I got a call from them telling me that he had been writing bogus deals, getting his 50% commission up front and did I know what was going on—oh yes indeed I did know. He also went by two names... *SLIMEY AND SLIMIER* and they found out that he was actually black listed by companies. *FOR A GUY THAT DIDN'T REALLY WORK HE SEEMED VERY VERY BUSY.*

Well when I told the parole officer about my ordeal that was enough for him to be called in as he was obligated to report every penny he received and since he took money from my mother and didn't report it that was all they needed, he had breached his parole conditions. A call was put out for him to come in for a meeting. He went in and acted as if nothing was wrong and his parole officer said that she had just been talking to me and on that note he went back to jail to finish out his sentence and was charged with more fraud to do with the company he was working for.

It was very stressful to go through all that but I have learned much from that experience and have moved on to much better things. I am currently in a very fun, happy relationship with someone that I trust, but I go through the same checklist each time I meet someone new. *CHECKLIST: HAS HE TRIED TO RIP ME OFF??*

—THE SLIME THAT CON MEN DO

More Creepy, Internet Slimes
—Anon.

Disclosure: What you are about to read is 100% true and not made up!

In October of 2005, I met a man on an internet dating site. He seemed reasonably sane, intelligent, and had a good job so after chatting via e-mail and telephone for a few weeks, I agreed to go on a date with him. This guy lived an hour away from me so we decided to drive our own vehicles to meet at a central location. We went for dinner first, which was pleasant enough. There were no "fireworks" to speak of, and conversation was limited at times, but it was our first meeting, so I wasn't too concerned. After dinner, he suggested we see a movie, since it was still early in the evening and the theatres were right next door. After the movie, he wanted to grab a coffee before heading back home, so instead of driving two vehicles to Tim Horton's I got in his car and we drove together. ***WELL IT ALL SEEMS SO NORMAL I JUST KNOW SOMETHING VERY BIZARRE IS ABOUT TO HAPPEN...LETS SEE.*** We went through the drive-thru and then he drove down to a park by the lake so we could sit and talk for a bit. Five minutes into our conversation, this guy suddenly turns to me and says "So do you want to touch my ****?" ***THERE IT IS!!!*** This is where you insert nervous laughter, which is exactly what I did, trying to hide my shock. ***I'M GUESSING HE ALSO WANT TO INSERT SOMETHING ELSE!!!***

After all, perhaps this guy had a weird sense of humour. He laughed too and said he was only kidding, that we would save that for our next date. ***OH SUPER.*** He changed the subject and starts talking about music, weather, the Blue Jays, whatever. Then he turned to me again, and said "Well why don't you just look at my **** then?" and proceeds to undo his pants. ***HOLD ON, ARE WE STILL IN THE DRIVETHRU? NO WAIT— I WENT BACK, WE'RE DOWN BY THE LAKE...***

My nervous laughter got a little more nervous. I was also getting really freaked out. ***NO KIDDING.*** Obviously this nut job was getting a lot of kicks out of making me uncomfortable. That part was very clear. Just as I was about to suggest this was not what I had in mind for a first date, he reclined the seat in his car and says to me "I wonder if there is enough room in this car to have sex with you?" ***GET OUT NOW... I REPEAT "GET OUT OF THIS CAR NOW"...*** This was when I said it was getting late and it was time to go. He agreed, noting he had to get up early in the morning and still had a long drive ahead of him. He drove me back to my car (praise the Lord), gave me a hug and a kiss on the cheek, thanked me for wonderful evening, and drove off into the night. *YOU ARE LUCKY AND HE'S THE SLIME THAT INTERNET NUT-JOBS, THAT OUT OF NOWHERE WANT YOU TO TOUCH THEIR PEE-PEES DO.*

Slimed By E-mail!
—Holly C.

I bet you already have some stories about guys dumping the girl via e-mail. *NOT SO MUCH.* That is what happened to me last fall.

I had been seeing this guy for a couple of months and thought everything was going great. *IT ALWAYS SEEMS THAT WAY.* He gave me all the right signals, I was falling in love and he had told me he was in love with me. He even made me a CD of love songs to listen to when he was away on long haul (he is a trucker driver). Well one day after one of his trips I got this e-mail out of the blue telling me he didn't want to see me anymore and that he wanted his e-mail to be the only explanation. *WHAT????* He didn't even have the guts to tell me to my face. I thought that was a pretty slimey thing to do considering we were even talking of moving in together. *NO KIDDING.* He had decided that he didn't want to be tied down after all because of his job. *YEAH, GOT TO BE FREE TO SLIME WHILE ON THE LONG HAULS ON THE ROAD TO...*   — THE SLIME THAT MEN DO

Have your own **SLIME ONLINE** story?

E-mail your story to **slime@humblehoward.com** and it could be included in our next book, *The Slime That Men Do 2!*

Here, make some notes, it could be therapeutic:

_____

_____

_____

_____

_____

_____

_____

_____

_____

_____

_____

_____

_____

_____

_____

_____

_____

_____

LOVE & LEARN

And Now Another In Our Series
"Chicks Are Slime Too... Well, They Can Be."
—Tim Miller

Just a quick one:

At the time I didn't realize it, but I was "the rebound" relationship for this, uh, lovely lady.

I had fallen hard and fast for her. She was beautiful, smart, had a great singing voice and so much more. (*SOUNDS LIKE KELLY PICKLER... WITHOUT THE SMART.*) In fact, she was the first girl I dated that I actually started having serious thoughts about marrying.

Well. We were working the same summer job (that I had helped her get) and happened to be working the same shift. During our lunch she dumped me. "Let's just be friends." "There's no one else." "Just need some space." All the typical dump-lines. And I still had to finish the rest of my shift with her!

Oh yeah, did I mention this part? It was my birthday.

Oh, and I can't forget to add that she was dating another guy three weeks later—who was in my band!! *LUNCH, BIRTHDAY, GOT HER A JOB AND SHE RAN OFF WITH THE BAND-MATE...*

—THE SLIME THAT CHICKS DO!

Slime in the Workplace
—Christine Burton

I used to moonlight cleaning houses and started cleaning for one of the guys at work. He's a divorced, part time father of two and in a management position. Anyway, shortly after I began cleaning his house (late 2000) we started getting close and sexually involved. *NOTHING TURNS MEN ON MORE THAN A CLEAN HOUSE.*

The relationship continued until the dreaded "L" word slipped from my mouth. That lead to numerous discussions and ultimately resulted in his attempts to put distance between us. *NOTHING TURNS SOME MEN OFF MORE THAN THE DREADED "L" WORD, OF COURSE THERE ARE SOME "L" WORDS THAT MEN LIKE, I THINK YOU KNOW THE ONE.* The reasons he gave were (remember these later on):

1. He didn't like the work/personal scenario
2. He wanted to step out of his comfort zone and
3. He felt that what he was doing was morally wrong (we weren't on the same relationship page).

At this point I gave him his key back.

Loser Boy, as I affectionately call him, left me a voicemail saying that he didn't necessarily want the house cleaning to stop and that we should chat. DUH!! *WOW…YEAH LET'S BREAK UP BUT WOULD YOU MIND STILL CLEANING UP FROM TIME TO TIME… WHAT AN ARSE.*

Now, another $2^1/_2$ years later, after many false endings it appears finally to be over. All this time he assumed that we'd remain friends—and if this story had a normal ending possibly we could have stayed friendly.

This is where the slime comes in. *WAIT, NOW IT GETS SLIMEY?* Not only do I get to see this slime everyday, I also get to see his new victim—she works here too!! (Remember Reason #1). I'm pretty sure he was playing both of us at the same time. She is well aware of the "history" we have.

Well!!! Doesn't he start up with the sexual innuendos on e-mail last week. We had a brief chat and I had to endure his pouty faces at my rejection to his "suggestion" for a get together. Doesn't he realize I could ruin his career and possibly his current relationship?? But that's just not my style. *HE'S LUCKY SHE'S SO NICE…*

—TOO BAD ABOUT THE SLIME THAT MEN DO!

Long Distance Slime
—Natalie Mitchell

I thought I would have nothing to contribute to this and now I have been crushed.

I studied abroad in Sweden just over two years ago for my final semester of university. While I was there I met a great group of French guys who I spent all my time with, one of whom I was dating. It was the love at first sight type of thing, he came to me from across the room, we didn't speak the same language, but we fell head over heels for each other. ***THIS HAPPENS TO FRENCH GUYS ALL THE TIME. MERDE.***

We were forced apart when our semester came to a close, but we refused to admit we were through. We said all of the typical things, made all the promises, and had lots of hope we might see each other again. This type of communication continued, to my surprise, for more than two years. I was always keeping him in the back of my mind, hoping there was a shot, knowing that if it weren't for proximity we would be together.

After much consideration I decided to fly to France to see if the sparks were still there. He was thrilled and invited me to his flat on the beach for a weekend, when I told him of my friends' doubts about us he argued that what we shared was beautiful. ***SOUNDS OKAY RIGHT? MAIS NO.*** I was thrilled, after so long we were finally going to give our relationship a chance.

I flew to France 12 days ago. Not only did our love affair cease to exist, he blew me off entirely. I flew to France and he didn't even have the decency to show up. In fact, he didn't even call me until the end of the week. No apologies, just excuses, leaving me abroad, alone, heartbroken and in shock.

This is the slime that men do. ***CEST TRISTE. LE SLIME DANS LES HOMME!***

Complicated Slime—But Worth It
—Sandi Huband

We'll call you Humble, him Not-So-Humble and me well, we'll call me Pie. **OKAY. I'LL BE HUMBLE.**

I have a girlfriend who owns a sex toy company, and she asked me to model her newest idea, and one of my favourites, her tickling panties on your show. Her real model backed out at the last minute and as a loyal friend I told her sure, I would help out, as long as I didn't have to talk on the show so I could not be identified.

My boyfriend at the time, Not-So-Humble, was extremely full of himself and kept me as his trophy girlfriend, he really never had intentions of something long term but I kept on hanging on hoping, as most women do, that I would change his mind. Thank goodness I didn't!

Not-So-Humble was a pilot of a major airline **COOL**. And, I have to admit, HOT HOT HOT. He took longer to get ready to go out than I ever did; he waxed more parts of his body than I have, and had a collection of cologne larger than the Bay's Beauty counters. **BUT HE WAS A COOL PILOT.** But damn he was sexy, very sexy.

When he found out that I was to wear these panties on your show he flipped. There was no way that HIS girlfriend was going to do this. The subject was eventually dropped. I slept at his house the night before the show, MISTAKE, because when my girlfriend called his house to ask what I was wearing, he got a little curious. He wasn't humble, but he wasn't an idiot either. **PILOTS ARE LIKE SUPER SMART.** I told him I had an important job interview and she was just curious about what I was going to wear. You know, chick talk. Not-So-Humble asked me about the show, and I denied that I was going to go ahead with it to avoid the inevitable fight, woke up at 6 A.M. and sped off to meet Madame Sex Toy Company.

All was going so well, there was no way Not-So-Humble could have known it was me on your show, none at all, I just wore the panties, and I thought if I moaned in a different tone than he was used to hearing, he'd never know. THEN, all of a sudden, your old partner says over the air "oh my God, it's a chick with a Habs tattoo on her hip." *MY OLD PARTNER DIDN'T LIKE THE HABS.*

We broke up over this. Because I wore a pair of panties that vibrated, I was dumped. I was heartbroken, but thank the heavenly skies above the panties weren't broken, they became Pie's very close friend until she eventually met her husband. *I'M CONFUSED. OH RIGHT YOU'RE PIE, SORRY.*

He doesn't wax anything aside from our cars. It must have been the uniform that turned me on to Not-So-Humble, but after the ride with Humble *ME?* And the humiliation Not-So-Humble put me through, Pie is very happy with Humble II (her husband) and would never ever dream of going out with a slimEEE character like Not-So-Humble again.

So, if a guy's stuff takes up more room in the bathroom than yours does, run girls, run as fast as you can, 'cause here comes the Not-So-Humble Man. This story has a happy ending, yours might not if you don't heed this warning!

PIE, ME, NOT-SO-HUMBLE PILOT, TICKLING PANTIES...SURELY A TALE OF THE SLIME THAT GUYS WHO WAX THEMSELVES DO!!!

Slime Told To Me...
Slime in Thunder Bay

This happened a couple of years ago. My first boyfriend, named John, went to university in Thunder Bay. After about four years of not seeing him or hearing from him, he phones me up and says, "Hey ya wanna come up this weekend for a visit." ***MAYBE HE DIDN'T KNOW THEY WEREN'T TOGETHER ANYMORE.***

Me being young and stupid I thought I'd go up and rekindle some of the things we had. So I fly up to Thunder Bay. It was a very last minute flight and so of course it cost a lot of money. I get up there and it's like Thursday, and he picks me up from the airport and I'm wearing this stunning outfit, you know... ***OF COURSE I DO.***

I'm looking good. So he helps me into the car and says "Are you hungry?" And I said "yeah." So we drive up to a drive-in window at McDonald's and he whips out a free French fry ticket... ***JUST FRIES, NO LITTLE BURGERS OR NOTHING.***

He was scrounging for pennies. He only took me there because he had a free coupon. Then he takes me back to his place and says "Well I gotta go to school." And then he leaves! He leaves me in his apartment with nothing to do and comes back about six hours later and starts watching a hockey game! ***THIS GUY MAY NOT BE SLIMEY, JUST A TWIT.***

At some point in the evening he turns to me and says, "I think you should go home." I'm like "Huh??" He said, "I think you should go home" I asked him why and he said it's not working out. ***MAYBE SHE WAS BUGGING HIM FOR MORE FRIES.***

I ended up at this seedy hotel and I'm going oh my God I have to pay all this extra money for the flight home. And a year later he phones to say hey maybe I should come up to Thunder Bay... ***YEAH 'CAUSE LAST TIME WAS SO MUCH FUN...***   —The Slime That Men Do

Slime in the Dictionary
—Wendy Birch

A few years back, I was in a relationship with a man whose picture appears in some dictionaries beside the definition of "slime." We had been dating about $2^1/2$ years and we were experiencing a bit of turmoil—mostly due to differing needs. I needed a boyfriend I could trust, and he needed more than one girlfriend. *YES, THOSE ARE DIFFERENT NEEDS.*

Things finally came to a head just before the August long weekend. He had been planning a camping trip up north with a buddy of his— and when something came up for said buddy, he assured me that he would go on his own—giving himself some good alone time to "clear his head." He promised to come back from his trip rested, and ready to be the "man I deserved" (his words, not mine).

And wouldn't you know it—the slime ball actually took another girl with him!!! He came back from his adventure—unaware that I knew of his foible—and actually suggested I come over and "bring my things so I could spend the night" (apparently he didn't manage to "get any" with the other broad!) *HER WORDS NOT MINE.*

But wait—it gets better! I decide to come over, wanting to find out just how dumb he thinks I am (just for the record, I'm the one with a specialized honors degree.) and he sits me down, wanting to tell me all about his "alone time" and how he's figured out just how much he loves me and wants to be with me, blah, blah, blah. Then, when I just can't take it anymore—he proceeds to lie right to my face when I confront him with the inside scoop!

Needless to say, it was the beginning of the end. He was literally up a creek without a paddle. Thanks for letting me unload. *LIES, SCOOPS AND PADDLES AND OF COURSE...*   —THE SLIME THAT MEN DO

Slime in the Dominican
—Jennifer Jesseau

I had been dating this guy named Steve, whom I met through my best friend's brother. I didn't know the brother well, but well enough to feel okay about hooking up with his friend. It was going so well at the beginning that Steve asked me to cancel a date I had with another guy. I really liked Steve and so I had assumed that at this point we would become exclusive. ***WHEN IT COMES TO SLIME ONE MUST NEVER ASSUME.***

About a month later, Steve had to go to Dominican Republic for a week for a wedding—my best friend's brother was getting married. This trip of course included my best friend, her mother and father and all of the extended family. Because I wasn't close to the brother, I wasn't invited. Steve made jokes about the fact that I wouldn't have to worry about him as my best friend and her entire family was going to be there to keep an eye on him. ***OH HA HA JERRY SLIMEFELD***

When he got back he called me on his way home from the airport. And twice after that to chat and to confirm plans for the weekend. It was nice to have him back and I looked forward to seeing him. He thanked me for all the little notes I left for him in his luggage and around his house. I missed him terribly but felt better that he was back safe and sound, and I was really looking forward to him meeting some of my family.

The next night my best friend Angela called. We chatted for a little bit about her trip but I could tell something was up. Angela sounded really nervous and said she had something to tell me and begged me not to be mad at her. I promised I wouldn't be mad. She told me she didn't like Steve and then proceeded to give me every last detail of an affair he had while staying in the Dominican. He had been sleeping with the bride's sister, also named Jennifer, the entire week. ***MAYBE HE'S ONLY INTO WOMEN NAMED JENNIFER***

Anyway, a few hours and a bottle of wine later, I called Steve on his cell phone. He was hanging out at a bar with a buddy. I pretended like nothing was wrong at the beginning. Steve asked me if I wanted to chat with his buddy Mike and I agreed. Mike got on the phone and asked me how I was doing.

"Mike, I'm not good."

"Why, what's the matter Jenn?," he said with honest concern in his voice.

I replied, "Steve didn't tell you?" I asked innocently.

"Tell me what?!"

I took a deep breath and with shaking hands said, "Mike, Steve didn't tell you that he spent the entire week in the Dominican Republic f**king the bride's sister?" Silence. Mike didn't know! *IMAGINE THE LOOK ON THIS DUDE'S FACE!*

I gave Mike all the gory details and he handed the phone back to Steve. I was calm but I told him exactly how I felt. He took it like a man. I also told him that he had embarrassed me in front of my best friend's family and that he was to call Angela and apologize. He did.

It was one of the meanest, most thoughtless things anyone has every done to me.

Even though we weren't totally an "item," it hurt my soul to think that someone could think that they could get away with that. And you know what Steve's big excuse was?

"I thought that what goes on in the Dominican stays in the Dominican. *DUDE, LAME. BESIDES THAT'S VEGAS YA TWIT.* "I can't believe Angela told you." Dumb ass. Did he really think a *best friend* isn't going to tell?   —THE SLIME THAT MEN DO

Slime... Short and Sweat
—Heather

I once dated a guy who invited me over to his house and proceeded to play video games. To make matters worse, while I was sitting beside him on the couch patiently waiting for him to finish, he reached over and wiped his sweaty hands on my pants without even lifting his eyes from the screen. To this day I don't think he realizes exactly why I broke up with him. *I CAN GUARANTEE IT.*

—THE SLIME THAT MEN DO

And Now Another In Our Series "Chicks Are Slime Too" A Sad One
—Shawn Glanfield

Amy and I met in school and were going out for over five years, I knew right from the start that this was the woman I wanted to spend the rest of my life with, and our families agreed. So on May 24th we went to Cullen Gardens I had paid to have my proposal done in fireworks at the end of the Victoria Day light show. It went off great and she said yes. *NICE TOUCH.* I was so happy.

We were busy making wedding plans when my mom was told she had cancer, so we moved up our wedding date so my mom would be around to see me get married. Mom was sent to hospital on August 1st and died August 6th. I spent the last six days with my mom in the hospital, and Amy was right there as well. My mom told the both of us how proud she was and even asked Amy if she would use her wedding ring for our wedding.

When my mom died I was a mess. We had three days of viewing before the service and Amy never showed up for any of it, she didn't call, show up or anything even for the funeral. Two weeks after my mom died I got a letter in the mail from Amy that said she didn't love me anymore and didn't want to marry me. At least I got my mom's ring back.

Just so you know women do slimey things too. *YES THEY DO...*

—THE SLIME THAT WOMEN DO

The Little Bird That Flew
—Jan Shah

Here's one for ya Humble:

I once dated a guy who was going through a difficult separation. His ex was a total lunatic—completely unreasonable, devious and even played the kids against him, needless to say it was a very stressful time. Throughout this period I was his grounding force—helping him to see the positive and get through the things that needed to be done—he called me his Rock of Gibraltar. *SO FAR SO GOOD RIGHT?*

In time, the stress of it became so much that he ended up going on Prozac, seeing a therapist and taking a leave from work. He was living in my small apartment by this time and we were talking about buying a house together and trying to get the kids away from his crazy ex. He gradually got better and announced one day that he had a bought a house in a town 50 km away and was planning on giving his kids 150% of his time so there would be no more time for me. *SURPRISE!!*

This was a complete surprise to me. I didn't even know that he had been looking at houses. I was devastated by his news and cried a lot of that time. He said he couldn't believe how wrong he was about me and my being his rock and that he thought I was stronger than this.

His therapist suggested I come to one of his sessions to talk about what I was going through. I was certain that I'd been pegged as a "Mothering Martyr" when he asked what I'd expected would happen after helping this man get better. My answer was simply that when you nurse a bird to health, you just hope that it won't shit in your hand as you're letting it go. *NOT UNLESS IT'S A REALLY SLIMEY BIRD.*

When this worm of a man left my apartment I didn't hear from him again. I did however find out that he started dating a 22-year-old only a few months after leaving me (he was 39 at that time). And finally to top off the sliminess, I swear this is true—he returned to England (without the children he so intended to devote his life to) only to start a relationship with his 17-year-old NIECE!! Yes—his sister's daughter— I kid you not! *BLIMEY...*　　　　　—The Slime That Men Do

Assault and Paper
—Tracey Lynn Bristow

A few years ago I was living with this guy. We had bought a house and as soon as we moved in together the FAIRY TALE began. I came home one day to find that the locks on our house had been changed. **WHAT FAIRY TALE IS THAT FROM? UNLESS THEY WERE GOLDY-LOCKS... SORRY.** I knocked on the door and the guy that I lived with told me to get off his property or else he would call the police. I thought that he was joking. He wasn't. The police came and gave me 10 minutes to get my stuff out of our house.

The problem, everything in the house was mine! So I could only grab clothes. The guy yelled and carried on the whole time I was in the house. The guy insisted that I was taking his stuff. I then showed the police my bras, underwear and clothes. They laughed. At this point I really didn't understand what was going on. I was thinking that he was mentally ill. Perhaps, on drugs? Met a new woman? **MAYBE ALL THREE, THE SLIME-FECTA. SORRY AGAIN.**

I really didn't know. I had to go the legal way to get the rest of my property. I served the guy legal papers to force him to appear before a judge to be told that I was legally allowed to go in the house to retrieve my belongings. I served him the papers at work where I thought that it would be safe.

Luckily he was outside when I pulled in. He freaked. He threw the documents at me and told me that he was going to call the police. I picked up the papers and shoved them in his hand. Then I drove home. Within an hour I was called by the police. They wanted to talk to me. I thought nothing of it. When I got there I WAS ARRESTED FOR ASSAULT!!!!! **NO WAY!**

Yes, it's true. I was handcuffed, put in a cruiser, drove to jail, finger-printed, mug shot, THE WORKS!

I had no one to bail me out so I spent 30 HOURS in jail. It was the WORST EXPERIENCE of my life. I read the court papers and it said that I was charged for ASSAULT. MEANS OF ASSAULT...

HIT OVER THE HEAD WITH PAPERS!!!!!! *THEY'RE DANGEROUS YOU COULD HAVE GIVEN HIM A MASSIVE PAPER CUT*

He had three of his buddies to back him up. This STUPID charge was SERIOUS. If I didn't get it dropped I would have had a REAL criminal record. After months of going to court (yes, months) I was finally able to convince the crown attorney to withdraw the charges. It wasn't easy or cheap.

One more thing, can you believe that the guy called me when I got out of jail and said "I didn't mean it"!!!!!!!

So that's my story. I've been HAPPILY SINGLE ever since.

—The Slime That Men Do

All's Well That Ends Slime
—Rosana Zammit

So I had been dating the guy Dave for over a year and a half and I was smitten. I knew he was the one and he gave me every assurance that he felt the same way. One day while passing by a jewellery store he suggested that we take a little peak inside. I was on cloud nine as I tried on engagement ring after engagement ring and Dave made suggestions about which he preferred. Over the next two weeks I spread the news of my impending engagement to my family and friends. I began to dream about my wedding and even selected my close friend Belinda (who had introduced Dave and me) to be my maid of honour. *SO FAR SO GOOD... BUT NO.*

Two weeks after taking me ring shopping we all went up to Belinda's family farm for a weekend away from the city. Dave and Belinda had always been close but I thought it was a bit odd when Belinda spent a fair amount of time running her fingers through my boyfriend's hair in front of me and the other guests. *MAYBE SHE WAS LOOKING FOR SOME-THING.* When confronted, Dave assured me that it was nothing and that any flirting was just a figment of my imagination.

Two days later Dave walked into my apartment and told me that he "couldn't see me anymore." It would seem that my "friend" whom I had selected to be my maid of honour had not been so honorable after all.

Soon after the break up I met with Dave to do the usual post-break-up exchange of personal items. During our long talk he admitted that he had feelings for Belinda (which I had obviously suspected), and then proceeded to seek advice from me, the person he'd taken ring shopping, about his relationship with the girl who was supposed to be my maid of honour at our wedding! *HERE'S SOME ADVICE DAVE, DON'T BE SUCH AN A-HOLE.*

As I believe in equality between the sexes I should add that Belinda's behavior was just as slimey as Dave's, if not more so. She not only got together with Dave and tried to hide it but she also did every-thing in her power to oust me from the circle of friends we had once shared. It was hurtful but also pitiful to watch: a girl succumbing to the ultimate level of sliminess and abandoning a long friendship for the sake of getting together with a slimey guy. *TOO TRUE*

Now this may be a tale of sliminess but these events have actually changed my life in some incredibly amazing ways. After crying, yelling and crying again about the revelation of the inner slime of two people I had loved and cared about I picked myself up and slowly started to rebuild... no... transform my life. My world changed and so did I. While I have and continued to stumble a lot along the way I have slowly grown in strength and confidence. Without undergoing the nasty and painful slime extraction process (as I like to call it) I might never have seen the pyramids, started singing again, applied for my Masters or had this opportunity to help fight breast cancer. I am living a life I otherwise would not have even imagined! So I figure, let slime be with slime, I'm too busy enjoying and appreciating my life in all its slime-free glory. *WHAT A GREAT ATTITUDE WHAT A GREAT STORY OF...*   —THE SLIME THAT MEN DO

Young Love Gone Slime
—Colleen McArton

When I was in Grade 8 this young boy I was dating asked me to go to the graduation dinner and dance with him. I of course said yes. So the night of the grad, he arrived at my house with balloons, flowers and a little graduation teddy bear. However, when we got to the hall, he sat with another girl in my class, let her wear his jacket when she was cold, and did not say another word to me all night. *THAT'S NOT NICE.*

Later in the evening, at the party my parents were hosting for my entire graduating class, he took me outside and broke up with me, saying that we were heading to high school next year and he just wasn't sure about our relationship, blah, blah, blah.

I later found out, through other boys in my class, that he really broke up with me because he thought I opened my mouth too wide when we kissed. *HE WAS PROBABLY A BAD KISSER ANYWAY...*

—THE SLIME THAT BOYS DO

Slime With No Spine
—Jen from Toronto

I recently finished dating a guy for three months who worked overseas and would be home for six weeks, then away for six weeks, then home for six weeks etc. When we first started dating he only had a month remaining on his 'home' stretch and we spent as much of it as possible together and everything was perfect. He even introduced me to his parents. Then he went away for six weeks, which was hard, but we e-mailed each other every day and spoke on the phone almost every day. He was just as attentive while he was overseas as he was when he had been home. *SOUNDS FINE SO FAR.*

When he finally got home within a week he'd gone from red-hot to luke-warm, but instead of breaking up with me he waited FIVE WEEKS until he had to leave the country again AND he claimed his employer had given him only one day's notice that his flight out was moved forward two days.

So, all of the sudden he called me in the morning and said he was leaving that day and would call me later from the airport.

Not only did he break up with me OVER THE PHONE FROM THE AIRPORT when he'd had plenty of time to do it in person, but he still didn't actually break up with me—he tried to make me think I was the one doing the breaking up! *NICE TOUCH* He said things like "I feel bad because I haven't been spending much time with you lately" and right away I thought "ahhhh... I see where this conversation is going!" but I didn't want to give him the satisfaction of making it easy for him because he was being such a spineless coward. I let the conversation continue until he had to resort to saying "well, what do

YOU want to do? Do you think we should put things on hold until I get back?" He actually had the nerve to try and make me believe he was concerned about what I wanted when what HE wanted was to make the break up official so he could get on the plane free and clear. He was too gutless to actually say it so in the end I did the dirty work.

So basically he left early, phoned me from the airport and made me do the breaking up. What a class act. *I THINK YOU ARE BEING SARCASTIC.*

Anyway it's the best thing that ever happened to me because it freed me up to meet the fabulous guy I'm with now. I am pleased to report that the new guy DOES have a backbone!

—THE SLIME THAT MEN DO

Slimey And Hungry
—Anon.

How can a guy come across so intelligent and yet be such a weenie? *I DON'T KNOW.*

I was dating this guy for a few months and he was totally commit-ment-phobic (married for 3 months previously lol) Anyways, e-v-e-r-y Saturday night was "guys" night and the "boys" would go out to drink and be merry. Which is fine and dandy, the only problem was I would get a call at 2 A.M.—not a booty call, but a call for me to pick up a sub and chocolate milk and bring it to him. *YOU'RE KIDDING.* Yeah, like that relationship is gonna last. *BOOTY WOULD BE MORE FUN AND LESS FATTENING.*

Anyway, I dumped him and gave him the local pizza place's number, hopefully that delivery guy gets a better tip than I did. *FUNNY AND SLIMEY AT THE SAME TIME...*   —THE SLIME THAT MEN DO

On and Off Again Slime
—Colleen Devoe

Here is my story about a man who is slime!

I have been in and out of a $7^1/2$ year relationship. We have had our problems but the one problem that has been consistent is my ex-boyfriend's old friend (who just happens to be a woman he was once intimate with). Last summer he broke up with me a couple of times after we had a fight. Recently he told me that one of those times we split up he went camping with this friend, just the two of them. He also told me that nothing happened between them and nothing has since he met me. He also told me that another time last summer when he broke up with me, he again went camping with this girl and a couple of friends of hers. Again nothing happened between them but he did receive some "oral" pleasure from one of her girlfriends. He asked me if I could ever forgive him. I told him that I could but only if he would give up his friend for good! He then said that he could not do this and I was being ridiculous just asking him. He also told me I was being inse-cure and paranoid. *EXCUSE ME, DIDN'T HE JUST TELL HER HE GOT A YOU-KNOW-WHAT FROM SOME OTHER CHICK.* Well I am not these things and have since ended it with him.

—THE SLIME THAT MEN DO

Vintage Slime
—Kathryn Burgin

Here is my slimey story. It's old slime, though. **OLD SCHOOL SLIME.**

Not to date myself, but almost 23-year old slime! It was my 17th birthday, and I was spending it with my boyfriend at the time, Rick. All went well (I thought), and he even bought me a cute little flower arrangement. I drove him home from north Burlington to east Hamilton Mountain—and I should mention that I did all the driving back and forth, and I don't recall ever receiving a penny for gas which is a big deal when you're 16 and driving a Dodge Royal Monaco—**THAT WAS ONE SWEET RIDE.**

Anyhow, when I got back home, I noticed a piece of paper in the chair he'd been sitting in, and I thought, "I'd better see what it is, in case it's important and something he needs." Well, it was a "you're dumped" note. **NO WAY!** On my birthday! **HAPPY BIRTHDAY!** He'd never even implied that we were on the outs, he acted normal the whole evening. He didn't even write the note himself; he had a mutual friend pen it for him (which I found out later—some friend).

Perhaps this wouldn't have bothered me so much, since he was a little bit slimey to begin with, but I lost my best babysitting job because of him. Still bitter? Just a bit, perhaps. **NO, IT WAS ONLY 23 YEARS AGO, MAY BE TIME TO LET IT GO … BUT STILL…**

—THE SLIME THAT MEN DO

Slime, Crime and Who Knows Where This Dude Is???
—Lisa R

I dated a guy in my mid-twenties who turned out to be Mr. Slime! He stole car speakers from a jeep and used my car as the get-away car! **THAT'S NOT NICE.**

So a couple of days later, I'm at work and I get a phone call from my dad, a retired cop. He tells me that there are two detectives at the house asking where they can find me. They explain to him what's going on, and that I should meet them at the police station right away! So I go to the police station, meet my parents there and have a 'little' talk with the detectives. **THAT SOUNDS LIKE ZERO FUN.** What I found out months later was that my dad asked a favor from the detectives, if they could put a scare into me so I would dump the boyfriend. Well I was scarred s**tless, **IS THAT A BAD WORD?** and dumped the guy! But who does that?! **YOUR EX.** Who steals something then uses their girlfriends car, so she gets nailed?! **YOUR EX** This guy is probably in jail somewhere right now! **IN JAIL WITH THE REST OF...**THE SLIME THAT MEN DO

Young Slime At Christmas Time
—Hayley Burch

I was preparing to go on vacation for Christmas with my family and had been dating a younger guy. Before leaving for my trip, we decided to spend some time together and do the 'Christmas' thing, i.e., exchange gifts. We went for a nice dinner, movie and then headed back to my place to hang out.

After saying good night he left and I finished packing and headed to bed. He called me not 15 minutes later saying he wanted to come back over if you know what I mean. **HE WAS HORNY.** He did and we continued to say good night. After quite a passionate encounter, while lying together I asked him if he was happy and well much to my horror, the answer was "well not really," **IT'S BEST NOT TO ASK,** "I don't think this is working out." I just lay there completely in shock, he asked me if I was alright and I just turned to him and said, "get out!!!!"

Needless to say I had to get on a plane this next morning with my family and spend the beginning of my vacation absolutely devastated. **I'M DREAMING OF A SLIMEY CHRISTMAS... HO HO HO...**

—THE SLIME THAT MEN DO

If It Walks Like A Duck It's A… Slime
—Lana

I was attracted to the President of the Christian club in my school, and my friend told me he was interested in me too. John (a.k.a. slime-guy) lived in Woodbridge and I lived in Brampton. Distance was what tore us apart and so our relationship amounted to three weeks of phone calls and three lunch dates.

One day, John decided to take me on a date in Woodbridge because he knew I hadn't been there in a while. The plan was for me to meet him at Yorkdale subway station where he'd pick me up. When the day came and I was on my way to the subway, John gave me a call. This was good, as I tried to call earlier because my parents just wanted to meet him and see who he was. After a long pause, he told me "Look… I've been meaning to do this a few days ago. I'm not ready for a relationship…it's not you, it's me… [pause]…" **OH MY GOODNESS NOT THE "IT'S NOT YOU, IT'S ME AHHHHHH!!"** For a while I tuned out because I was in shock. I didn't see this coming so soon.

ANYTHING would have been better than the It's-not-you-it's-me-routine. **NO KIDDING.** My only reply was: "well, better it be done now instead of later [sob,sob]." He then adds, "I hope this won't affect your membership/position on the Christian Club?"…I began to cry even harder, to which he responded by hanging up. Picture it: all dressed-up in the heart of Toronto and I had nowhere to go. And to think, if I had gone to Woodbridge he would have broken up with me there and I would have suffered an hour car ride home. **BOO THIS GUY**

We held a Pub Night one Friday night. I came fashionably late thinking I would be the only girl from the club who was to attend. To my surprise, I saw two tables: one with a bunch of my fellow-execs in the club and another with John and his guests. These guests happened to be all girls. When I went to sit down, he introduced the girls sitting across from him. They seemed like nice people except, I was wondering why one of them gave me a blank stare. I decided to sit at the next table where I was comfortable with familiar faces. My friend on my right notices new guests coming in and decides to introduce us, "This is Lana, Matthew, Mark, Luke, and John... and John's girl-friend beside him"..."my heart starts racing*...did he say 'girlfriend'??? *I THINK HE SAID GIRLFRIEND!* But wait. There wasn't anything to be angry about. It's not like I ever wanted to be with him, AGAIN. Why should I be angry? Angry? Me? Me, angry? NOT AT ALL.

Meanwhile, I was contemplating throwing a tantrum and slapping my shoe across his head. *VERY UN-CHRISTIAN-LIKE BEHAVIOR.* How-ever, I was saved by sheer generosity from all the guys around. They were nice enough to buy me all the drinks I wanted. So I did a good job of keeping my cool. Little did I know that my emotions would take over the next morning, when I was suffering the worst hangover IN THE WORLD!! *BOO HANGOVERS.* The man didn't even have the decency to introduce this girl to me as his own GIRLFRIEND!!!

The above offences were committed by the same slime-guy. Names were changed to respect the actors involved. Ladies, if he smells like slime, spends your money like slime and wastes your time like slime, he is a SLIME-GUY. Perhaps by divine intervention, I'm hoping some insight will still restore my faith in slime. *YOU-KNOW-HOW-MOVES IN MYSTERIOUS WAYS BUT NOT WHEN IT COMES TO...*

—THE SLIME THAT MEN DO

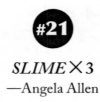

SLIME × 3
—Angela Allen

Humble, I have three stories to tell you about the slime I've dated.

1. I accepted a date with this well-spoken, well-dressed man. He takes me to a dive for some drinks and in the middle of drinks he gets a phone call and announces he has to leave. Why? I ask. He then tells me that he's a drug dealer and needs to make a "deal" to pay for our night out. *WHAT A CATCH.* He then left me there and two men in their late '60s hit on me, sending me into tears. Luckily I knew the bar owner who drove me home.

2. Last year I had to have my tonsils taken out and my boyfriend at the time dropped me off at my mother's (who was going to look after me) he kisses me goodbye, tells me he loves me and that he'll call me the next day to see how I'm doing. I get home from the hospital all drugged and in pain. He calls me and dumps that day. *REALLY?* The worst part about it is that because I was so drugged up, my mother had to tell me that I got dumped after I got well. *I'M CONFUSED YOU GOT DUMPED BY YOUR MOM? KIDDING.*

3. I was dating someone and it was getting semi-serious. It had been six months at this point and we were making plans for the next couple of weeks and all of a sudden he falls off the face of the earth. I found out through friend weeks later that he had won a contest. He won a lot of money and took off without even telling me. Four months later he finally resurfaces because he ran out of money. *IF YOU ROLL ALL THREE OF THESE GUYS INTO ONE YOU'D GET SOME KIND OF SUPER STRAIN OF...*

—The Slime That Men Do

I Could Write Your Whole Book
—Monica Marquis

It is true, I have attracted my fair share of slimey men. In fact, I think that I have taken quite a few for the team. Ladies, you can thank me. *I'M SURE THEY DO.*

Take Slimey B, a real charmer. I was totally in love with him, thought we were getting married, New Year's was approaching—we were at a large dinner party and the hostess addressed Slimey B across the table and asked him when he is leaving for Mexico. *HUH?* He left the next day with his ex-girlfriend. Slimey! But it gets better.

He steps off the plane and comes right to my house! *LET'S HOPE HE GOT THE RUNS.* But the ultimate slime experience was this: For a full year I had so many penis encounters in public places that I was ready to kill the next guy that decided to flash me. *EXCUSE ME.* This happened to me in Toronto, in the daylight, on the subway, on the streetcar, on the street with cars whizzing by. One guy had the nerve to approach me and walk right past me as he masturbated. *HE DID NOT!* The guy on the subway was having a party with his penis at 9 A.M. and I rang the alarm. *PARTY'S JUST A FIGURE OF SPEECH I'M GUESSING.*

Oh and then there was the loser who was in the phone booth talking to someone (his wife?) and as I walked by he plastered his whole body against the glass and tongued the glass... ugh *SORRY 'BOUT THAT I WAS JUST TRYING TO BE FUNNY...*

Then, my boyfriend's daughter asked me if I was her dad's girl-friend. I said what do you think? She said I think so, because you are the one who is here the most. *KIDS CAN BE SUCH CUTIE PIES.* I met my boyfriends other girlfriend. I didn't know it until I told her who I was, and her face dropped. I think he told her about me, but she must have thought I was some old frumpy thing that he hung out with in his spare time. *I'M ASSUMING YOUR NOT FRUMPY, BUT THESE MEN SURELY REPRESENT...*   —THE SLIME THAT MEN DO

Sleeping in a Tennis Court!
—Alison, Toronto

My boyfriend of three years promised to come to my place one night after he finished a couple of drinks with a friend. He called from a payphone at around 9 P.M. saying his cell phone battery died, but he was finishing his last pint and would be leaving momentarily. *A POST-PINT BOOTY CALL?*

When 10 o'clock came and went along with 11, 12 and 1, I finally decided to go to bed after leaving many worried and frantic messages on his dead phone. The next day I received a call from my boyfriend around noon explaining that after deciding to drink until last call, he thought going to an after hours club was a good idea. *OKAY.* Then, instead of taking a $15 cab to my apartment, he thought it was more fiscally responsible to sleep in a public tennis court! When he woke up, he took the train home to his mom's house, even though the infamous tennis court was a five-minute walk from my workplace.

Although he never understood why I was upset, he felt guilty enough to beg me not to tell his mother what happened! Needless to say, this boyfriend quickly became my ex-boyfriend, but his legacy remains in that my friends and I still refer to being really drunk as 'sleeping in a tennis court'! *FUNNY, SAD AND ANOTHER TALE OF...*
—The Slime That Drunken Guys Do

One Slime, 3 Strikes
—Anon.

There is a guy I dated off and on for over a year. We work together. That's already two strikes I should have paid attention to: Never go back to someone you already broke it off with and never date someone at work.

The last time we got back together it was great. He came to family functions and got along great with my siblings. We even went on a romantic one-week getaway together. I had fallen in love. *AWWWW.*

After the romantic getaway, he became detached and distant. I didn't know what to do, so I wrote him a letter telling him how I felt about him. The next day he started laughing and being childish because I confessed that I love him — I was so mad that I said I didn't want to talk about it. It hurts when you put your heart out there, only to be laughed at. *TELL ME ABOUT IT.*

He continued to be distant, and a few days later, a co-worker of mine who didn't know the guy and I were seeing each other, came to my desk to tell me she caught the guy looking at engagement rings online. I was so happy that I told a friend, and she sat me down to tell me she over heard that the ring was not for me. I confronted the guy and he said it was my fault. *HOW?* Because I chose not to talk to him about the letter I gave to him, he asked out an old flame and decided they should get married. I was stunned. *WHAT A DICK.*

So yes, the guy wooed me back for the last time with full intentions of marrying the girl his mother arranged for him. *HUH!* Getting closer to my family and going away on the romantic getaway was all part of his plan to have one last "fling" (for lack of a better word) before he got married. He's happily married now… strike three, I'm out. *YOU MAY BE OUT BUT'S HE'S A BATTER COVERED IN SLIME…*

—THE SLIME THAT MEN DO

"Lieutenant Dan is a Slime"
—Melissa Jarrett

When I was in my last year of university I met this guy who I was instantly attracted too because I thought he looked like Gary Sinise, *THE "CSI"/"FORREST GUMP" DUDE!* Who I had always found to be attractive. It should have been a clear warning signal when I met this guy, that this was going to be a strange relationship, when he didn't drive… at all… didn't know how… didn't care to learn… so right from the start I drove everywhere… but sometimes you over look the little oddities because you are just so attracted to the person. *NO KIDDING, ASK MY WIFE.*

I started to notice that he always had the worst breath imaginable. Like something rotten. For my birthday he got me a used version of a Disney movie from the video store where he worked, in VHS… not even the DVD. Didn't wrap it or give me a card. Just handed it to me. *ROMANTIC, BAD BREATH, BAMBI…*

Anyway, to get to the slime—about four months into this bizarre relationship (I could go on and on) I had to get my wisdom teeth removed. I have always had a bad reaction to being put under and knew that I would be very sick. But since he couldn't drive he couldn't take me to and from the dentist, so I was home alone, sick. He then *e-mailed* me to tell me that he would be going away for the weekend to a friend's cottage. He even mentioned that the friend was a girl and that the cottage was a real roughing it cottage, no TV, nothing to do, and that he used to really like this girl—but told me it was no big deal. Right. No big deal, because I always go on romantic secluded week end getaways with former crushes and that's normal. *OH SURE, SURE DOESN'T EVERYBODY??*

I didn't even wait for him to get back, I dumped him through e-mail. I know that's bad, but… there was also no phone at the cottage. *BUT THERE WAS E-MAIL!*

But it didn't end. I couldn't get rid of him. He kept sending me e-mails, but weird e-mails about his sexual dreams, and our wedding. He even sent me an e-mail telling me that he went to a dentist and had 9 cavities. *THAT WOULD EXPLAIN THE BREATH.* I didn't respond to a single message but they kept coming like we were having a conversation. I would block him and change my e-mail but somehow he found my new e-mails, and he would write more letters, and show up at places where I was meeting people. *OKAY, NOW HE'S GETTING CREEPY.*

I quit my job because it was in walking distance of his house. I called the police, and showed the letters, and they thought this was pretty bizarre as well and spoke to him, telling him to leave me alone. *NOW HALITOSIS BOY IS GETTING DOWNRIGHT DANGEROUS.*

I really thought it had stopped. Six months went by, I moved to another city and one morning I checked my NEW e-mail account—and found a note from him! I sent the nastiest reply I could come up with and have not heard from him since. I can't watch anything with Gary Sinise in it anymore without cringing. *NOT EVEN CSI?? I HEAR IT'S QUITE GOOD…*   —The Slime That Really Creepy Guys Do

Story about a Slime Ball
—The one who got revenge.

I slowly got involved with a co-worker after knowing him for about a year. I was his boss. Company policy did not allow co-workers to date, so it was even more exciting that way. We will call this guy James. *OKAY.*

James was a very interesting guy, with a bit of mystery to him. He never really talked about his family or anything, which we all found kind of odd. I just thought he was a private person. His brother would sometimes stop by the office to chat, but that was about it. No one really knew anything about his personal life. *MAYBE HE WAS A SPY?*

One day, he came to me and started to talk about his home life. He seemed upset and depressed about something. He started to talk about how he lives with his mother and stepfather, in their basement apartment with his girlfriend. *EXCUSE ME?*

This was the first time any of us had heard about his girlfriend. He mentioned how depressed he was feeling about his relationship. He wasn't happy and no longer wanted to be with her. He just didn't know how to handle kicking her out. They had been together for a very long time and his family adored her.

He told me that he was supposed to get married the following month in Cuba. He did not want to go through with it. I told him to do what would be right for him and left it at that.

The following month came, and he told me he had finally broken up with her. However, he still needed the vacation time he was supposed to have taken in order to get married in Cuba. He said he wasn't able to get a refund on the tickets and that he was going to take his buddy with him instead. (He told this to at least 17 co-workers).

We hooked up about a month after that. We dated for about a year. *OH, ALL THAT OTHER STUFF HAPPENED BEFORE YOU "HOOKED UP."*

To make a long, long story short, I found out that he did actually get married in Cuba and his whole sob story was just a cover so he would be able to cheat on his wife with me. *YOU'RE KIDDING!* Not only is it bad enough to cheat on your wife, but to cheat only a month after getting married? When I confronted him about what I knew, he tried to give me every pathetic excuse like "I only married her for money" or "I need her financial support because I'm in such debt" or anything he could possibly say. *WEREN'T THEY SHARING A BASEMENT APARTMENT?* He *really* didn't want to get busted for this. He said anything he could, from "I love *you!* Not her!" to "I'll leave her as soon as I can!" This guy was a real piece of work. With all the lies and fabricated stories, you would think he was a writer for a soap opera. I fired his ass. Keep in mind, this guy planned this whole charade from the get go, waited months for it to pan out and who knows how long he would have let it go on had I not found out! That is what you call a slime ball. It still makes me sick to this day when I think about all the trouble he went through just to get laid by someone other than his wife. *WOW.*

So, that was that. Can you believe a human like this exists? He seriously needs help. He's sick and perverted.

Does the wife know about all this? Of course she does! I wasn't going to let him get away with something like this! She had a right to know, don't you think?

It really bothered me though, to know I was going to be responsible for turning this poor girl's life upside down. I thought about it for a while but I was so infuriated that nothing else really mattered other than getting him busted. I thought about how I would do it. I had to do it in a way that would show proof, so he couldn't lie his way out of it. So, I put together a little package that would be sent via mail straight to his house. Inside this package, was every note, card, picture and letter he had ever given me. The letters were very obvious, hand written and there was no denying he was involved with another woman. The wife was going to see that these weren't written to her! They did not have her name on them.

Just as I suspected, she ended up getting the letter marked "confidential" with his name on it. Like any other curious wife, she opened it and that's how she found out. I described in the letter to him how he made me sick and how I didn't want anything he had ever given me. *HOLY MOLEY!!!*

She never called. I did receive a call from James though. He was screaming and crying on the phone, saying how much I ruined his life. I just laughed to myself because he ruined his own life.

So, Slime-ball finally got was coming to him and I couldn't have been more pleased. I wonder if he has learned to play in his own yard instead of jumping over the fence and dirtying someone else's. *LET'S HOPE SO...*   —THE SLIME THAT MEN DO

A Slimey Guys Confession
—Former Slime Ball

I'm not proud of it, but I was slime once. *I'M LISTENING MY SON.*

I was talking to this girl from Lethbridge, Alberta in a chat room one day and we hit it off immediately. Now, I wasn't in the room trying to pick up a gal, we just connected. We continued to chat every day for about two or three months when we finally exchanged phone numbers. We would talk for hours on end at work, at home, even when we were at our friends' houses. *YES, YES GIRLS ARE NICE.*

One day while I was at work, she called me from a travel agency, asking if I was interested in going to Lethbridge for the weekend so we could finally meet and spend some time together. I thought it was a great idea, but I couldn't really afford it at the time...She said she would buy the ticket and I could pay her back whenever. So I said sure! *HMMM I DON'T LIKE WHERE THIS IS GOING.* She ended up sending my ticket via FedEx along with a picture of herself. You know how you get a picture in your head of someone when you just hear their voice? Well she didn't look anything like I thought. To be blunt, she was the same size as me! But I thought it would still be a nice trip and we could have a great time together, after all we clicked so well. *OKAY...*

I was to be staying at her sister's apartment, with her and her sister. To make a long story short, we had a great conversation during the two hour drive from Calgary to Lethbridge and when we arrived at her sister's house, well, her sister who looked more like the image I had in my mind before I received the picture. *OH DON'T TELL ME.* Her sister and I hit it off so well that we ended up sleeping together that night, while the one I was supposed to be seeing was in the next room. I ended up spending all weekend with her sister instead of her, except for the drive back to the airport, when she asked me when I was going to pay her back for the ticket. My response to that was, "when I come back to visit your sister." *YOU SLIME-BALL!*

I never ended up going back to Lethbridge, never saw or spoke to either of them again and couldn't track her down later to pay her back when I realized what a slime I had been. *GEE HOW DID YOU FIGURE THAT OUT...*

I hope all the slimey men out there realize what they're doing actually hurts people... I did... just too late that's all. *GOOD BOY, NOW FOR YOUR PENANCE TAKE THE MONEY YOU OWED THE ONE SISTER AND GIVE IT TO THE BREAST CANCER FOUNDATION...*

—THE SLIME THAT SOME MEN USED TO DO!!!

That Gift Looks Very Familiar...
—Katie

Here I go spreading some slime.

I had a wonderful and beautiful boyfriend. We had been happily dating for years before his true colours came shining through. *THAT CAN TAKE TIME...*

A few days before Christmas we were shopping together and with arms full of bags we roamed the mall in festive bliss. *MY FAVOURITE KIND OF BLISS.* Our shopping had concluded for the day, but before we left I had one little item that I wanted to pick-up for myself—mini speakers for my Walkman (Hey, I told you this was a while ago!) *I REMEMBER THOSE THE WERE LIKE iPODS ONLY NOT REALLY.* I picked out the pair that I wanted and paid for them (around $15⁰⁰) *THAT WAS A WHILE AGO* and we headed our separate ways.

Once I got home and began to sort out the gifts that I had bought for everyone, I realized that I didn't have the speakers. Later, on the phone, I asked him if he had them in his bag and he said he did and that he would bring them over the next time I saw him. *THINGS SEEM COOL SO FAR.*

Skip ahead to Christmas morning when my family and I open our gifts. I anxiously opened my gift from my sweetie (which he had left under the tree the night before) only to find that he had kept and wrapped those speakers and given them to me as my gift. *COME ON, NOT THE ONES YOU HAD PICKED OUT AND PAID FOR??* That was it! Speakers that I had picked out myself and PAID for, he had the nerve to wrap up as my gift. To make matters worse, when I called him and asked him what he was thinking, he didn't see anything wrong with what he had done. All he said was "But, isn't that what you wanted?" *SLIME GUY LOGIC.*

Needless to say, that was the end of us dating. I was so profoundly hurt by him doing that that I have rarely ever spoken about it but I still have those speakers. They sit loud and proud, plugged into my MP3 player, kept as a reminder of just how slimey men can be!

—MORE OF THE SLIME THAT CHEAP GUYS DO

Slime With A Married Guy
—Valerie

Several years ago, I began dating a guy from work (yes a terrible place to start!) He was having problems in his marriage and was separated from his wife. This probably should have been my first clue; however, he basically swept me off my feet! *SOUNDS GOOD BUT NO...*

I couldn't believe that a guy could be this into me! Where had he been all my life! So for several months it was amazing. He was out of his house, staying with friends and yes, sometimes even with me. I thought he was moving on. But as the months progressed, he started missing phone calls to me and even schedules dates and visits. All the while giving me excuses that something came up and the ex was causing problems for him. *OH THAT EXCUSE.* He of course was trying to 'nip it in the bud' so to speak, trying to keep her at bay so he could get out of the marriage clean or so he kept telling me.

So months turned into two years! I know what you're thinking— what was I thinking????? *ACTUALLY I WAS THINKING ABOUT SOME SOUP BUT I'M BACK NOW...WHAT WERE YOU THINKING?* Broken promises, too many to count and a broken heart over and over again. But I kept thinking she was the problem. Making things difficult for him to move on, a bitter women! I literally thought this man was my soul mate. Even though he would break my heart over and over again, but when it was good, it was awesome and somehow that kept me going.

Well, all good things must come to end! I finally caught him. The final straw was a date to move in together. That came and went without a phone call and I was heartbroken. I began to really do some digging. And now, in retrospect, I don't know how I didn't see what was always in front of me! *I THINK IT'S EASIER TO SEE IN THE REAR VIEW SO DON'T SWEAT IT.*

For all these years, he was with his wife! I'm not even sure if in the beginning he was separated! He never had any intentions of ever leaving and I had been totally blind and felt utterly ridiculous! *YOU SHOULDN'T HAVE HE WAS THE ASS.*

It's been over two-and-a-half years now since the 'truth' finally became clear. A slime ball is one that can lie day in and day out and eventually even believe the lies he's telling! He was leading a double life, the ones you see on TV or read about in books! *A LOT OF THEM ARE IN THIS ONE!*

You'd think it wouldn't be possible in real life but he did an exceptional job!

He definitely deserves top honors for being a "slime ball!!!"

THE SLIME THAT MARRIED GUYS THAT SAY THEY ARE LEAVING THEIR WIVES BUT LIE JUST TO SCREW AROUND DO.

#30

No Time For Summer Slime
—Anon.

I met Rod in January of 1999 through an introduction service. We dated for a few months and then as summer approached, he decided that he didn't have time for me in "his summer." *?????* We decided to stay in touch and in November we got back together. *?????*

I knew his employer was not doing well so when he told me that he was going to be taking some time to visit his friend in New York City and spend the rest of the week traveling in the U.S. looking for another job, I didn't think too much of it. *I'M STILL WONDERING WHY HE COULDN'T SEE YOU IN THE SUMMER.* I did think it was weird that he would take a trip like this without an agenda. (Sometimes women are way too blind!)

When he came back he took me to dinner. When he picked me up he had a CD holder in his SUV that was made from two Hawaiian license plates hinged together. *WEIRD.* I looked at it and said that I thought it was neat and asked him where he got it from. His response was "there." I said "where, in Hawaii—when were you in Hawaii?" His response was "last week!" *WASN'T HE SUPPOSED TO BE IN NEW YORK??*

He then went on to tell me that the trip had been booked before we got back together and he didn't want to lose me again, so he made up the story. This is his other story:

He had free flights with points that he had collected from his American Express and his "friend" had a time share in Hawaii, so it only made sense. It was a once in a lifetime opportunity and they were "just friends!" I later found out that he dated this "friend" in the summer while he didn't have time for me! *AHH HIS SUMMER "FRIEND"*

Being extremely naïve (or stupid) I bought his story and continued our relationship. In November of 2000, I gave birth to a beautiful little girl and stayed with her father until February of 2003. *WHAT YOU CAN'T SEE IS MY HEAD DOING ONE OF THOSE CARTOON DOUBLE TAKE THINGS ALONG WITH THAT EYE-YI-YI TYPE OF NOISE. HAWAII, NEW YORK, SUMMER, BABY…IT'S ALL TOO MUCH TOO FAST AND OF COURSE TOO SLIMEY…*

—THE SLIME THAT MEN DO

Short, To the Point and Slimey
—Anon.

My boyfriend and I had been going out for four years. He started cheating on me. He was going out with another girl for seven months before I found out. He would only see her once a week and when he did he would tell me he was working overtime. Anyway, to make a long story short. *VERY SHORT.* The day I found out he sent me 100 red roses. I guess he was feeling a little guilty. *YA THINK?* When I finally talked to the other girl she didn't know about me either and I asked if she ever just dropped by his house because he had pictures of me around the house. She said when she went there he had pictures of her and her kids up. What a slime. *HE SLIMED BOTH OF YOU...*

—THE SLIME THAT MEN DO

Picture, Perfect, Slime!
—Lani

While I was in college I worked part-time at a clothing store at a mall in my small town. I ended up meeting a guy who came in and we started dating. He was a little older than me, I was 19 at the time and he was I think 27 or 28. I fell head over heels for this guy; I thought he was the be-all and end-all. I mean all through high school I didn't really have a lot of boyfriends, *ME NEITHER* so for this older guy to take interest in me and want to date me, made me feel awesome. *SEEMS COOL SO FAR*

So everything was going well. We dated for about five or six months, and then of course he started acting a little weird. One day I came home from classes and my mom said that there was a letter for me that had been dropped off in the mail box. I went up to my room to read it and enclosed was a "break-up" letter and a *picture* of the two of us that was just taken two weeks before, all happy and cuddly! *A PICTURE??? WTF?*

First of all, this older, mature guy doesn't have enough guts to break up with me face to face and than on top of doing it in a letter; he encloses a *picture of the two of us*!!! *AGAIN I SAY WTF?*

I was completely devastated, but just to show how much more mature I was than he, the following day I went to his apartment to pick up all my stuff. Conveniently he wasn't home, just his roommate was, but I acted like it didn't bother me and I told him to say hello to my ex and walked out the door.

WOULD YOU LIKE TO CLOSE WITH A MESSAGE FOR ALL GUYS…

Message for all guys out there, please do not breakup with a girl in a letter, we deserve a whole lot more than that!!!! *AND I'LL ADD DON'T DO IT WITH A PICTURE…*   —THE SLIME THAT MEN DO

Air, Sea and Slime to the Rescue
—Jean Stewart

Hi Humble. *HI JEAN.* I want to share this story with you.

I fell in love with an amazing, handsome, kind, athletic man who was with air and sea rescue out of Trenton. He had two phones, with one if it rang or the pager went off he had to leave immediately as there was an emergency. I learned from him what to do if I fall into the ice, amongst other survival tips. He could never really talk about the rescues as they were confidential. *OH YEAH, NATIONAL SECURITY STUFF, FALLING THROUGH THE ICE OR WORSE, RUNNING OUT OF ICE!*

I was with him eight months—when He "disappeared" over Christmas and into January. Then in January, my mom died suddenly. I was devastated and called, went round to his house, nothing. I finally sent him an e-mail. *BAD SIGN.*

Six weeks later I bumped into him. He tells me his is so sorry and was testing some aircraft in Vancouver; they were under security and could not take calls to give away the position—plausible right?? *SORT OF, OKAY.*

Anyway we got together again for a while... till he disappeared again. I later found out that this guy worked in the local automotive factory on the line. *SEARCH AND RESCUE AT THE AUTOMOTIVE FACTORY?* The calls were from other woman, and he obviously WAS around in January, probably didn't want to show his face in case his cover was blown!! He was stringing along another 3 woman at least, and is probably still doing so!! *WOW, SLIMEY AND ENERGETIC.*

As I'm writing this the reality off all that time kicks in and I cannot believe anyone could be so callous—a definite slime-ball!!! *DEFINITELY... THE SLIME THAT GUYS WHO PRETEND TO BE SOMETHING COOL AND STRING THREE CHICKS ALONG...DO*

What Not To Say in Response to "I Love You!"
—Jill Robinson

Well, were do I start. A few of us girls were sitting around one day talking at work and came upon the topic of expressing our feelings to the boys we were dating at the time. The other two did so, and one of them now is married to that guy and the other still keeps in touch with her guy. I, on the other hand, was devastated with the outcome of my situation. *HOW BAD COULD IT BE??*

I called the "Boy" to tell him I'd like to see him that night. We meet up and we are sitting in my car and I finally get enough nerve to tell him how I feel and the conversation went something like this.

Me: I really need to tell you how I feel about you; I think I am in love with you.

(Lots of silence) *BAD SIGN*

Him: So!

Me: (Sitting there with a shocked look on my face)

He turns to me and says: What! Are you gonna drive yourself off a cliff now or you gonna be ok? *OH THAT'S HOW BAD IT COULD BE.*

Me: Is that all you have to say?

Him: Yup

NOT EXACTLY THE STUFF OF ROMANCE MOVIES.

And he got out of my car and I never saw him again. **WOW.**

—THE SLIME THAT MEN DO

Let's Go Away So You Can Slime Me!
—Melanie Serjeant

A few years ago I was dating this guy, (who happened to be my best friend's brother) who told me he was taking me on a surprise trip and to book the time off work. **A LOT OF THESE STORIES SEEM TO START OUT WELL AND THEN...** As it got closer to the time to leave we were only talking to each other maybe a couple times a week and hardly saw each other. **THINGS WERE ALREADY STARTING TO SOUR.** So the day arrives and we were off to the airport he told me we were going to Cuba. Until then I had never been on a plane before so I was super excited. We got to our seat and I asked him if I could have the window seat. He told me he was really tired and wanted to sit there so he could use the window as a head rest. I felt like Drew Barrymore in *The Wedding Singer*. **UH, OKAY...**We arrived at the hotel and went through the introduction thing and finally got to the room. I snuck in the bathroom and put on a slinky sexy outfit and came out. **MUY CALIENTE!!! ARIBA.** Right then and there the butt hole broke up with me... **I'M SORRY??** The butt-hole broke up with me the first day of our vacation!! **WOW.** Needless to say we spent the week in complete silence. Not one word spoken between the two of us. **MAY I SAY WOW AGAIN.** It was just horrible. When we got back to our airport we went separate ways. **WHAT THE HELL HAPPENED?? WHY DID HE DO THIS?**

It took me awhile to get in touch with my friend but when I finally did she told me the whole story. Apparently not long before we were to go on our trip he wanted to break up with me, but didn't because our tickets for the trip were nontransferable and he couldn't cancel without loosing his money. *WHAT AN ARSE.* So his plan was to stay with me until we came back from the trip. I guess that's why we hardly spoke or saw each other as much before we left, and probably why I didn't get the window seat. *THAT, AND THE FACT THAT'S HE'S AN ARSE!*

He told my friend (his sister!) he couldn't hold off once he realized I wanted sex.

I think this was the worst thing that has ever happened to me. *THE SLIME THAT GUYS WHO TAKE CHICKS ON SURPRISE TRIPS TO CUBA AND THEN BREAK UP WITH THEM DO!*

Hey, You're Doing My Slime!
—Deborah Read

About 10 years ago I met a guy we will call "Scott."

Scott and I met on the job and quickly entered into a torrid relationship based mostly on, well I admit it… great sex. After several dates, I moved in with him *DATES, WOW YOU KIDS MOVE FAST.* As the months passed, I suspected he was cheating on me—and in particular, I suspected he was cheating on me with another much older woman who worked in the same company. On Valentine's Day, we made the usual plans for dinner and drinks for 7 P.M. and I rushed home to get ready. The clock ticked away to 7:30, 7:45, 8:00, 8:15—finally at 8:30 and still no sign of Scott, I was done waiting and I left our apartment only imagining where he was and with whom.

I took streetcars and buses all the way from the apartment we lived in on Lakeshore, through downtown Toronto and to my sister's place in Scarborough, all the while crying at the sight of lovey-dovey couples on the street holding hands having the most romantic of Valentine's nights. *LIKE ONE OF THOSE ROMANCE MOVIES WHERE THE HEROINE GOES LOOKING FOR SCOTT TO HAVE MORE GREAT SEX WITH.*

At around 9:30 that night Scott started calling around looking for me. My sister refused to tell him I was at her house. The next morning at work, the very woman I suspected he had Valentine's dinner with was in our office coffee room talking loudly in my earshot on purpose about where she and Scott went the night before, all the great gifts she got from him, and the great time they had. I was devastated, hurt and angry at the same time. I lived with the guy and she went out on Valentine's with him!! *I'M A LITTLE CONFUSED...WHY WOULD SHE TALK ABOUT THIS IN FRONT OF YOU?? DID SHE SUFFER FROM ITCHBAY DISEASE?*

Now, though she and I worked for the same company, our offices were separated by a two-storey tall gangway in the building complex's atrium—very scary to walk across if you're afraid of heights. Later that day, as fate would have it that she was walking across alone at the exact moment that I was—I met her in the middle and had serious words with her, to put it mildly—I did not lay a hand on her, but I guess she felt a bit afraid because the whole incident happened on this precarious gangway. A couple hours later, I got called into HR and was fired for threatening another employee! *NO WAY.*

BUT... this sad Stupid Cupid story actually has a great ending, because later that very same day, I met the person who would later be my husband, while crying in my coffee in the restaurant in the atrium—we have been happily married for 10 years. In addition, after being fired from the job, I started my own company which is also 10-years-old this year and going strong. *WOW, THINGS HAPPEN FAST IN YOUR WORLD, CONGRATS ON THE DUDE AND THE BUSINESS... BTW HOWS THE YOU KNOW, UH FORGET IT...*

—The Slime That Men Do*!!!*

Shortest Slime Ever
—Anon.

For my birthday, he bought me a pack of cigarettes—the small pack—and two of them were missing. —The Slime That Cheap Smokers Do

More Slime Told To Me—the Slime Conspiracy

I had been seeing a guy for about three years. His best friend was also a good friend of mine and we always hung out and stuff. My boyfriend had to go away on business and suddenly, his best friend starts hanging around when he's not there. *JUST YOU MAKING SURE YOUR OKAY?* Yeah. He keeps coming over every night, and I was starting to wonder what he was up to—but of course nothing happened. *OF COURSE.*

My boyfriend returned and next thing I know he's acting like he's really mad at me. And I was wondering what's going on. And I said "Well, what's wrong?" And he said "I know you slept with him." *WHAT?* He said he knew that I had slept with his best friend, and his best friend had told everybody, all of our friends in our crowd, that I had slept with him. My boyfriend believed him over me, and he left me. *COME ON... DID YOU EVER CONFRONT THE BEST FRIEND?*

No, because I never I heard from him again. As soon as my boyfriend left, well his friend went with him I guess... *ARE THEY HAPPY "TOGETHER"?*

They probably are. They deserve each other.

Here's my theory. My boyfriend went away, did some nasty things up wherever he was, the reason his friend was hanging around was so they could start the rumour so that when he got back, he could dump me! *I CONCUR!! THE SLIME THAT MEN-FRIENDS DO*

Very Bizzare Slime
—Anon.

Okay, basically, I was seeing this guy for a few months and he had always told me about his brother from Italy. After a night shift I went over to meet my guy in the morning for coffee, and this young man answered the door and said, "Uh, Sam's not home so why don't you come in and just wait for him?" ***BELLA BELLA. I'M GUESS THIS IS THE BROTHER FROM ITALY.*** Right, and this is eight in the morning.

So I'm waiting, talking, just small talk, I mean, I just met the guy. We were upstairs in the TV room and he uh, sits down beside me, starts making some weird "moves" on me. I was a bit uncomfortable but he said "well, we'll just watch TV." ***DIDN'T WE JUST MEET THIS DUDE?***

He said "Boy, my brother's taste really changed, you're beautiful, you're so young." ***HE KNOWS YOU'RE GOING OUT WITH HIS BRO...***

But he perseveres, it doesn't seem to matter if I was dating his brother, he's trying to get intimate... ***OKAY.*** He's right beside me, getting the arm a bit around me... and so I said "Well, I should get going." Then he says, "Oh no, we'll just watch a movie." So at eight o'clock in the morning he popped in a porno movie. ***NO WAY.*** And it wasn't even at the beginning of the story, it was right in the middle of something. ***NO WAY TIMES TWO!***

Yeah. The brother of my boyfriend want to watch porn with me at 8 A.M.! It's like he thinks... "The way to a woman's heart, of course, is a little coffee in the morning and a porno film." And he doesn't even start it at the beginning. ***WHICH IS SO IMPORTANT WITH THOSE MOVIES CAUSE YOU MAY MISS SOME PLOT POINTS AND THEN THE WHOLE THING MAKES NO SENSE.***

So I get up and said "Just tell your brother I was here this morning." I called my boyfriend at work and told him what had happened and he was like, oh that's just Tony being funny. No big deal. Well it was a big deal to me and a while later we broke up, not just because of that but believe me it didn't help. ***THE SLIME THAT WEIRD GUYS THAT WANT TO WATCH PORN WITH THEIR BROTHERS GIRLFRIENDS AT 8 IN THE MORNING DO.***

Three Part Slime
—Rita

There's three slimey parts to my story.

First, while I was in school in the US I was dating an American guy, and during the summers I would come back to Canada. Finally after two years, I decided I would go home that summer tell to my parents I was moving in with him. **NO SMALL STEP.**

Yeah. So I broke the news to my parents two weeks before I was on my way back down to school. They pretty much freaked and I stopped talking to my mom for those two weeks. Five minutes before I was going to jump in my car for the 28-hour drive back down to school, the phone rings. It's my boyfriend.

He says, "I don't love you anymore, I want to break up with you, and find your own place to live because I cheated on you." **NICE... WHAT ABOUT PART 2?**

Okay so I drive down, I'm a mess. We still have the same circle of friends, so we did run into each other quite a bit. One good friend, Jennifer, really helped me through it and made me realize what a slime he really was. When I graduated we're all saying our goodbyes, and my ex is bawling, telling me how much he loves me. So we kept in touch for the month or so until I get the phone call he's now going out with Jennifer. **THE SAME JENN WHO HELPED YOU IN YOUR TIME OF NEED?!**

Okay, now part 3: Now Jennifer and my ex are going out. **WOW.** Now they don't want to talk to me anymore. Four months go down the road Jennifer decides to break off with him. So he starts calling me to find out how he can win Jen back. **THE OTHER CHICK?? THIS GUY IS UNBELIEVABLE.** This goes on for about another month—you know, maybe I can put a good word with Jen so she'd go out with him again. Finally he calls me one last time to tell me that he's not interested in Jen, he's interested in me and would like me to move back down there so maybe we can plan a future together. **UH, NO NOT SO MUCH...**

—THE SLIME THAT MEN DO

When Irish Eyes Are Sliming
—Grace

Well this happened in Ireland, when I had been going out with my boyfriend for one year. It was my going away party; I was going off to Canada. We were at a bar, and I was with my friends, and one of my best friends Caroline was there. We had a few drinks... *WOW, THEY HAVE BARS IN IRELAND TOO?* Then my boyfriend just decided that he wanted to go the bathroom, so that was fine. Then we're chatting away and Caroline says "I'm just gonna go to the washroom." So she was gone for a while, and about fifteen minutes later, I realized that she had been missing for a while. *YOUR BEST FRIEND CAROLINE?* Yeah. I went to the washroom to see if she was there but I couldn't find her so. I was just walking by a big large window in the hallway and I looked out and saw John's car. *JOHN YOUR BOYFRIEND.* John was my boyfriend. The door was open, so I thought maybe somebody was trying to break into his car or something. So I went outside, and Caroline and john are in the car making out. *OOOPS. YOUR BEST FRIEND.* Yeah, and my boyfriend for a year, at my going away party. Well I went back to my friends and we decided that we'd, you know, get the bill, which was quite expensive, and leave it with him, so we all went outside. So we stood around the car, and I knocked on the window. *YEAH.*

Yeah, I just knocked on the window and he rolled it down and I threw the bill at his face, and I said "when you're finished, how would you like to take care of this?" *NICE GOING AWAY PRESENT...*

—THE SLIME THAT MEN DO

Too Good To Be Slime
—Anon.

I met this guy and fell in love with him right away. He was perfect in all senses—very good looking, he had money apparently, he said his foster mother had died and left him some land, he had a beautiful car, my family liked him and everything was perfect. We actually moved in together right away. **SOUNDS PERFECT.** It was too perfect. And I was young and naïve. Apparently he was a brick layer, he was laid off at the time and he was waiting for his unemployment money. So we were living on my credit cards, going out all the time having fun, and I started getting suspicious after a couple months, when no money came in. *AH HA NOW IT GETS SLIMEY.*

We rented a car one weekend and ended up having a fight because I was getting suspicious. I asked: "where's all your money?" And so on. Then he took off with this rent-a-car and I was upset, it was in my name, I paid for it. Anyway, a couple days later at work I get a call from a relative of his, and she said that there was a death in the family and did I know where he was. And it turns out—well she said to me, she said "Did you know that this guy is married?" *WAIT A SECOND... HE WAS MARRIED?*

Honest. Apparently he's a compulsive liar; he did this often to his wife where he would disappear for weekends, but never two months in a row. His friends didn't even tell me that he was married. Good friends, and so I had no idea. *THAT HE WAS A SLIME-BALL.*

No, well finally, I put an A.P.B. out on him for my rent-a-car, and his wife and I waited at the car rental office for him. The two of us were on each side of the door so we could surprise him. *NICE LITTLE STING OPERATION.* Yes. That's just what happened. He pulled, he had another girl in the car with her two kids, and he was gonna take care of her—a stripper he had met at some bar. *WHERE DOES HE GET THE ENERGY???*   —THE SLIME THAT MEN DO

Slime On The High Seas
—Anon.

About a year ago my friend Anne and I went on a Caribbean cruise because we figured the only slime there would be stuck to the bottom of the boat. We needed a holiday and figured we'd meet some nice guys. *OKAY.* So we're at this formal cocktail party of the captain's. One of the cruise staff, Scott, introduced himself. Very nice guy, decked out in a tuxedo, seemed pretty classy, no slime showing.

About three nights later we were at the nightclub on the ship and Scott came in, a little drunk. ***SOME DRUNKEN SAILOR.*** He has my friend on one side of him and me on the other, and we're just watching everybody and he turns to me, and without Anne realizing it he says "I'd really like to take you down to my cabin." Well no, no, I just turned him down; I mean I barely knew the guy. Little did I know, he turned to around my friend and asked Anne the same thing. Within seconds of me turning him down he asks my friend if she would like some action. *A LITTLE NERVY.* Basically. So I had to leave the room, I mean at this point I thought I would laugh right in front of him. When I came back they were dancing. No big deal. I sat at our table to wait for them when Anne came off the dance floor with a look on her face like she's seen a ghost. I asked her what was wrong and apparently he had, on the dance floor, in front of a lot of people, just looked at her and said "Would you take that dress off?"

—The Slime That Cruise Ship Men Do

Slime Out Of The Closet
—Linda

Okay, this is about an old boyfriend, and we were very serious. I thought I knew him quite well, and one night when he told me that he would call me the next day I knew something was up because he usually calls me when he gets home. So I drove to his apartment, and I waited, and finally about 2:30 A.M. I see a cab pull up. He got out and started coming up the walk. I glanced away when I looked again I saw a girl follow him. *SO YOU ARE INSIDE THE APARTMENT LOOKING OUT THE WINDOW?* I didn't have enough time to leave the building without being seen, so I went into a storage closet in the hallway. *LIKE IN THE MOVIES.*

Now here is the slime of all time, okay. While I was in the closet, he called my house and left a message: "Hi honey, I'm just missing you very much. I thought I'd call to see how you are." *SOME PRE-SLIME GUILT.* So I waited long enough, but not too long if you know what I mean. But I thought they would go in the bedroom, but they didn't. They stood right outside this cupboard. So I waited just long enough so it wasn't too embarrassing, and I opened the door and popped out. *WOW. WHAT DID HE DO??* He grabbed me, as if I was going to do something to this girl. I mean I felt sorry for this girl. At this point it's 4 A.M. and he says to her "get out." So I said "Don't worry, she's not leaving, I'm leaving." And that was that. —THE SLIME THAT MEN DO

Sweet, Silent Revenge on a Slime
—Jennifer Ringham

I dated this guy about 17 years ago. I was attracted to bad boys at that time. I figured at least he had a job! But, he also had a problem with being faithful. I stuck it out for too long thinking I would save him and he'd realize I was the one for him. *GOOD LUCK.* I wasn't—thank God!!!

It was normal for him to stay out all night and come home with some dumb ass excuse, I would buy it just so he wouldn't leave me, although I knew better. We lived in a small town and there were just too many rumors flying around about him. *I GREW UP IN A SMALL TOWN TOO AND I KNOW WHAT YOU MEAN...THERE WAS RUMOUR THAT I SLEPT WITH A LOT OF CHICKS...WHICH I STARTED!*

The final straw was when he arrived home in the morning, his usual 7:00 A.M. and of course I had, had another sleepless night wondering who the feck was he with now. *I'M GUESSING YOU MEAN THE OTHER "F" WORD* He had scratch marks all over his back, which he said came from someone's bike that was hung in their garage. *YEAH RIGHT!* That bike sure had long nails!!! He was hung over and I said no more.

I let him crash out and proceeded to plan his day for him when he would finally awake. *CUE THE EVIL MUSIC* I knew his routine and carefully and quietly set him up. When he got up I was already gone. But first, I loaded his blow dryer with baby powder. *YES, YES.* He had his shower, blow dried his hair and the powder turned his hair into dough!! *(EVIL LAUGH)* Then he had to have another shower, dried his hair and then put hair spray on it to style. Ha Ha. I dumped his hair spray and put lemon honey cough syrup in it. Hence, he had to have another shower. (He later accused me of peeing in it, I guess I would have, but I never thought of that.) *DRATS, YES I SAID DRATS—MORE EVIL LAUGHTER.* I knew he would want to play some solitaire, while watching a game before he would go out prowling that following evening. Damn, I took the remote and the receiver with me and the cards to boot. If he wanted to watch TV he would have to get up and turn the channel himself and without the receiver, he only got 13 channels. *MOOOHA-HAHAHAHAH IMBECILE* I even took the toothpaste with me so he's have skanky breath on his next night of pick up some poor drunk victim-chick.

Oh well, he's gone now. My friends still laugh about it when reminiscing, and still refer to him as "Double FL" Feck Face Loser!! *I'M GUESSING AGAIN YOU MEAN THE BAD "F" WORD AGAIN.* Awwwwwwwww, the sweet taste of silent revenge!

—THE SLIME THAT MEN DO

#46

Mr. Right Until The Next Slime Comes Along...
—Anon.

A friend of mine gave me number of a guy who seemed to have the perfect package for me: fun, outgoing, outdoorsy, and attractive. He seemed to be the real deal and we had started out incredibly romantically. He was from out of town so we spent a week on the phone for at least five or six hours a night, and I felt like I had met my soul mate. *WOW.* We did the same things, had the same interests and even though he already had children, he wanted to get remarried and would have more. Needless to say I was HOOKED. *I'M HOOKED.* To drive it in further, he suggested that, assuming there is chemistry, he could see us getting married.

Well I was four weeks from my fortieth birthday and that kind of whirlwind romance was just what the doctor ordered. But then a friend called me and told me to watch out, he was a player with all the right moves but in the end wouldn't stick. I thanked her for her warnings and then did what every "I haven't given up hope" woman would do. I said to myself it will be different with me. And he did have all the right moves. *REALLY! LIKE WHAT?* He surprised me at the airport. I was coming back from a business trip and he wasn't meant to be home until the next day... but there he was (we had exchanged digital photos through the week and was waiting for me as I came out of customs— right out of every girls dream—okay, he didn't have a white horse.) *I DON'T THINK YOU'RE ALLOWED TO BRING THOSE INSIDE.* He greeted me with a great big hug and said those magic words: "You are even more beautiful than your photo." Needless to say, the first week was terrific and we quickly fell into a nice pattern.

A month later came spring break. I was off with friends and he with his family, but he was meant to be back in time for my birthday. *SO WHEN DO THINGS GET WEIRD?* Well, there was a dinner planned with friends on the Saturday of my birthday and he said he was too tired to come to dinner, having just returned from a trip. I bought it and was so happy when he actually showed up for twenty minutes. The next morning he was meant to come for brunch with my parents. Let's just say his laundry was more important and he showed up late. *UH OH* Again excuses and a bit embarrassment. I was confused but was still having fun celebrating my birthday and as it was a big birthday, I had more celebrating to do. The next Saturday we had dinner with friends and I ignored his seeming disinterest. Well it turned out the "dinner" was actually a huge surprise party with friends, an amazing evening filled with funny stories and laughter. *NICE.* How special I felt, surrounded by amazing friends full of love and laughter and this great guy. Well, by the end of the evening it was clear that his attentions seemed elsewhere. When he was too overwhelmed to bring me home, my girlfriends warning started flashing bright. *SLIGHTLY.* Then next day I called it off. I called a close friend of mine to tell him and he said "oh I am so thankful, I didn't want to tell you on your birthday" but it seems "the player" had asked a friend of his out on the Friday before the party. The end result was the same, it seems it wasn't different with me at all. I guess my time was up and he was ready for the next in line. *THE SLIME THAT VERY, VERY INSECURE MEN THAT KEEPING GOING FROM WOMAN TO WOMAN BUT WILL EVENTUALLY END UP ALONE DO*

Short, Strange and Slimey
—Amanda Chard

Well every good man knows that women are very self conscious, and it takes some courage to wear all those outfits they love so much that make us sexier. *ME TOO!* I was with my ex (you will see why he is my ex) and we had had the perfect night—we'd gone out to a romantic dinner, we were giggling and talking about everything, and I thought nothing could ruin this. *OKAY.* Well, I was wrong. We got home and I assumed were going to have a little fun to conclude the perfect night. *FUN IS GOOD.* I headed upstairs without him to change into something very sexy and called him upstairs to view. I am standing there trying to look my best. He entered the room, looked at me and said

"What are you wearing that for?" *HE DID NOT!* He did! Well this started an explosion. I gave him the look of evil, and he still didn't get it, he just walked away and said "Nice, ok, I'm going to watch TV while you get changed." *NICE.* It took a lot for me to get in the crap, and it was only for him, not me. We argued and did not talk for three days and a week later we broke up.

—THE SLIME THAT MEN WHO DON'T GET "IT" DO.

Male Nurse, Slime-Messenger
—Danielle Carriere

I dated a male nurse last year who told me that he was working on obtaining a visa so he could go to the U.S. to get his masters degree. He said that he would be leaving when the paperwork was finalized. I wanted to meet his parents but he always made an excuse. They were working, out of town, busy. I felt like I was being "hidden" from them, so I said that if I wasn't good enough to meet the parents, then I wasn't good enough to hang out with. *MAKES SENSE.* He told me that he had fallen in love with me and that he didn't want to lose me. He brought me flowers, left a stuffed animal with the security desk at my apartment, and showed up in the middle of the night professing his love for me. *SOUNDS GOOD... SO WHAT WAS SO STRANGE?*

The strange part of this relationship was that his preferred method of communication was cell phone text messaging. I told him that I would prefer if he would just call me, but he rarely did and always used text. Then he announced to me that his visa had come through and that he would be leaving. I was shocked. Then, I didn't hear from him for a few days so I called and left a message on his voice mail for him to please call me. I got a text message back saying that he was at the gate waiting to get on the plane and needed some time to think. I was like, "WHAT?????" I text messaged him back to call me. The final message I got from him ever, by text message, was GOODBYE.

——THE SLIME THAT MALE NURSES DO

Mexico Time Share Slime
—Anon.

Everybody who's heard it says this is a classic. Sad part is, it's all true. So, without naming names, I'll give you the low-down. *LET'S HAVE IT THEN.*

I dated this guy and he told me that he needed a week alone to focus on his four children. I said, "of course." He told me that he would call after the week was up. I said that would be fine. After not hearing from him for a week and a half, I decided to call him. He wasn't home so I left a message on his answering machine saying that I was concerned about him and if he would please give me a call. *NICE SHOW OF CONCERN.* I heard nothing for another two days. My mother had met him while and thought he was a great guy, and she was worried as well and decided that she would give him a call. Still no response. *NO RESPONSE FOR MOM??* Mom was worried and decided to give his parents a call. His father said something to the effect that he thought his son and I had broken up and that his son was currently away on vacation with his new girlfriend who he'd been seeing for about three months. *OH REALLY, HOW WEIRD WITH THE PARENTS GETTING INVOLVED??* My mother was shocked and my ex's father apparently was as well. *ME TOO!* When my ex got back, he telephoned me and left a message on my answering machine that his father had his facts mixed up, there is no other woman and that we need to get together as soon as possible to talk. *SURE, SURE, LET'S DO THAT!*

As it was quite late when he left this message, I didn't return the call because I had to work in the morning. When I got to work, he was waiting for me at the elevators and asked if we could talk now. I told him to meet me after work and we could talk then. He was very nervous but agreed to meet me after work. At this meeting, I asked him about the woman his father was referring to and he said that she's "just a friend who I went to high school with" and that his father was reading more into it. *OH YEAH THAT OLD EXCUSE.* I asked him why he hadn't called me after a week like he said he would, and I asked him how the four children were doing. He said, "uh, do I look a little tanned to you?" I said, "uh, I guess so." He told me that he had taken a trip to Mexico just to get away. ***WHY TAKE THE OTHER CHICK THEN??*** He said that he went with this "friend" but that she paid her own way and it was strictly on a friend basis even though they slept in the same bed in order to get a cheaper room at the resort. ***WELL THAT MAKES TONS OF SENSE.*** The ex begged me to believe him and that nothing happened between them. I gave him a second chance and our relationship continued for six months until I moved to another city. We kept in touch by telephone and he flew back for a visit in the fall.

On one of the visits he said, "Sweety, I have to confess something; it's about that Mexico trip." I was waiting for him to admit that he had actually been physical with the other woman. Then to my complete astonishment he asked me if I knew what a "time share" was. I told him that I didn't. He said that it's a contract that people enter into to guarantee use of a particular property in Mexico at any time of the year for as many years long as the contract is for. I didn't know where he was going with this, so I said, "oh, you bought a time share in Mexico?" THEN, to my COMPLETE HORROR, he admitted that yes, he had bought one WITH THE OTHER WOMEN, a contract for 25 years!! ***IT WOULD HAVE BEEN BETTER IF HE HAD SLEPT WITH HER!!!!***
—THE SLIME THAT MEN DO

The Newspaper Slime
—Marilyn Regendanz

We met in Halifax some 20 years ago. I was divorced and coaxed into going downtown partying with the girls. An attractive "gentlemen" by the name of Mark came up and we struck up a conversation. ***OKAY.*** He was from Toronto, worked for a large, well-known newspaper, and was in the midst of being transferred to Halifax. He was trying to meet/make some new friends. I had recently moved back to Halifax from Toronto so we had something in common.

We chatted for hours until the bar closed. We exchanged phone numbers and spent the next few evenings together. He was charming, interesting, attractive and I enjoyed his company. I had asked the usual questions during our conversation marathons. After I got to know him a little better, I asked him why he was still single and hadn't settled down. He gave me the standard "just haven't met the right girl yet" answer and added "until now." **OOOOH DREAMY.**

He had to go back to Toronto for a couple of days to attend a friends wedding. He apologized profusely, hated to leave but plans had been made months prior to go to this wedding with a buddy of his. We made a date for Sunday evening. Tuesday came and I hadn't heard from him. I got worried. He'd been so punctual. I thought he would have called if something came up. I called the Toronto newspaper and asked for him. I was put through to his secretary who was very helpful. He wasn't in but my heart relaxed when I knew he was OK. But then, disappointment set in that he hadn't let me know of a change of plans. I asked her if she knew if Mark was coming back to Halifax and she informed me that Mark and, I'll call her, Sue had flown back Sunday. I hung up the phone dumbfounded. *???????* My mom came to visit me at work and I told her the story. She said something sounded fishy.

Curiosity got the best of us. Later that day I called back and spoke with his "very helpful" secretary again. I posed as an old high school friend working on a school reunion. **GOOD SPYING.** I found out all kinds of interesting things about Mark. Not only was Sue his wife, she was his *second* wife. **NO WAY!** They had gone to the wedding on the weekend and then flown to Halifax. I guess it's hard to call a potential girlfriend when you're wife is with you. **IS IT?** He called a couple of days later. I didn't mention what my investigation had uncovered. I told him how worried and disappointed I had been. He apologized and asked how he could make it up to me. I told him to make reservations at the best restaurant in town. I thought I would ask him more pointed questions. I decided to order a meal that would slide into his lap easily if he continued the lie. I asked him point blank if he'd ever considered marriage or actually been married. He said no. I was poised to drop my dinner in his lap but my mother's words rang in my ear telling me how inappropriate it was to make a scene in public. Besides, the meal was excellent! *MMM FOOD GOOD... MMM FREE FOOD BETTER.*

We went back to my place and settled on the couch. He kissed me and told me how much he had missed me. So, I asked him how the wedding went. After he finished, I asked him if his wife enjoyed the wedding. He faked a very good quizzical expression and said "what wife"? I replied with "You know. Her name is Sue." I told him where they were married, that it was his second marriage, his first wife's name, that he wasn't actually being transferred to Halifax, as well as some other details. *WOW, YOU ARE AWESOME.* I told him that he didn't have to lie and that we "could have" been friends. I also told him that I could have introduced him to other people in Halifax. We could have enjoyed each others company, as friends, provided he'd been up front with me and honest with his wife. He apologized repeatedly and begged my forgiveness. I told him to get out of my apartment and that I had no time for liars. He called repeatedly over the next few days. My final words to him were that I was naive not stupid!

THE SLIME THAT MARRIED GUYS WHO ARE TRYING FOR SOME SIDE-ACTION DO.

Another Mr. Right Turns Into Mr. Slime
—Marlene Huffman

I've been told over and over that you should never put all men in the same category. Well. I met a guy and dated him for about five months. I thought long and hard about getting into the intimate level of our relationship and decided to go ahead after much encouragement of his love and commitment to me. *NICE.* It was my birthday and he invited me for a romantic dinner on a Saturday night. We had a wonderful dinner and evening, ending with making love and confirming our love for each other. We woke early to the sounds of our puppy wanting to start the day. *DO YOU MEAN REAL PUPPIES OR IS THAT CODE FOR*

LOVE RELATIONS... NEVER MIND... at 7 A.M. the doorbell rings and a dark-haired lady pushes her way in, carrying two coffees and sits herself down at the kitchen table. My love says in a real quiet voice please do not make a scene I will explain everything later. *WTF?????* I am the most patient person who has always worn my heart on my sleeve. I was just too uncomfortable and needed answers like who are you, etc. *SLIGHTLY!!!* I walked into the kitchen and introduced myself and asked where she met my man. Well, she was a little set back and my man asked me to join him in the other room. I excused myself and we looked at each other and all he said was please do not make a scene. *I THINK A SCENE IS ALREADY IN PROGRESS...* As I was about to be sick I expressed my anger in a way that this lady could hear. I proceeded to go back and talk a little further. She said she met him a while ago on a dating site. I was crushed but held my composure, she said what the heck is going on? I said sweetheart we have both been *had.* She threw the chair, walked around the table gave me a big hug and proceeded to call the man every word that is not allowed to be heard publicly. She stormed out the door shouting that you involved my kids you (*bleep bleep bleep*) I got dressed and proceeded to leave and all he could say was he screwed up and he loved me. *TOO LATE.* It took four weeks before he finally stopped calling, after my quiet threats of harassment charges. I have now given thanks to this man for adding yet another block to my wall and it will take much time and trust to ever be in a relationship again. *SORRY TO HEAR THAT... BUT ITS NOT YOU IT'S...*

—THE SLIME THAT A-HOLES DO.

Campground Slime
—Jacki

Now, you've probably gotten a lot of stories about cheaters and being cheated on. This one's got to be at the top of the slime list. *BELIEVE ME, IT'S QUITE A LIST!*

It was the May 24 long weekend and I was unable to make it to our campground the first night because I had to work late, so my boyfriend headed up without me. The gang that night consisted of my boyfriend, two of his friends and two of my girlfriends. *EVERYTHING ALWAYS SOUNDS FINE, THEN...* I made it for the last two nights of camping. The weekend went pretty well, although I was getting a weird vibe from my boyfriend and one of my girlfriends. I found out later that instead of being satisfied that I would be there the next night, my boyfriend decided he needed some lovin' on Friday night. So my boyfriend and one of my girlfriends apparently slipped into the woods and did the nasty. *LET'S HOPE HE GOT A RASH IN HIS NASTY AREA* Oh, does this not sound so bad? Did I forget to mention that it was our first anniversary that weekend? *I'M GUESSING THERE WON'T BE A NUMBER TWO!!!*

—THE SLIME THAT CHEATING CAMPGROUND PEOPLE DO.

#53

Slimed By a Guy Having a Whiz??
—Lori M.

Behind our office there is an alleyway that is very well used as many companies back onto it. So, of course, there are always plenty of people back there before and after work and at lunchtime using it as short cut to get to work. At the end of my work day I was leaving the office and, unfortunately, saw a man peeing off to the side in a little parking lot. He was not a street person because he was wearing khakis, a dress shirt and a man bag. *HE HAD A MAN BAG AND YOU SAW HIS... FORGET IT... ANYWAY...* I assume he was coming home from work. As this is not the first time I have had the pleasure of seeing this, I averted my eyes and continued down the alley. He finished his business and as he came out to the alley he realized that I must have seen him.

"Sorry lady, sorry." he said.

I smiled, broke eye contact and continued on my way.

However, he must have thought that some sort of dialogue had been established because he said:

"So how was your day?" *WOW, THE PEE-GUY IS VERY SUAVE.*

"O.K." again I broke eye contact and continued walking (get a clue buddy).

But that didn't discourage him, for he continued on with his one-way conversation. Finally, he said: "You're a pretty lady but you must be married. Let me see your ring finger." *WTF??* At this point, I was just blown away. How could you think that any woman would want to have a conversation with you never mind contemplate dating you when she has just witnessed you peeing on a wall? *SOME GUYS WOULD.* What excuse could you have beyond being too lazy to find a regular wash-room? A side point: I have never, ever, seen a woman peeing in the back alley.

P.S. This is not a good opportunity to pick up a woman. Who wants to relate the story to friends/family—oh, we met when I saw so and so peeing in the alley. How could I resist? *HOW COULD ANYONE...*

　　　　　—THE SLIME THAT GUYS WHO PEE IN BACK ALLEYS DO

Have your own **LOVE & LEARN** story?

E-mail your story to **slime@humblehoward.com** and it could be included in our next book, *The Slime That Men Do 2!*

Here, make some notes, it could be therapeutic:

_____

_____

_____

_____

_____

_____

_____

_____

_____

_____

_____

_____

_____

_____

_____

_____

_____

_____

_____

_____

MARRIED SLIME— 'TIL SLIME DO US PART

Ring Around the Slime
—Natasha Wilson

First I would like to say that I love my husband and have obviously gotten over what he did enough to marry him last fall—though I'm not fully over as I felt the need to e-mail my story.

SLIME YES, BUT NOT BAD AND APPARENTLY MARRIAGE-WORTHY!

My husband and I have been together for 11 years. In our sixth or seventh year it was no secret that I would like to have an engagement ring. So, at Christmas, there was a small box-shaped present saved for me to open at my parents' home. I knew this would not be the ring that I so desired (we simply couldn't afford it being university students) but I thought that maybe he would give me earrings or some other kind of jewelry. I opened the present with my entire family present. Inside the box there was a small velvet container. When I opened this container it was in fact a velvet ring box. But—instead of a ring inside there was piece of paper sticking out of the slot the ring would have sat. The piece of paper simply read *"You Wish."*

NICE TOUCH!!

I was so angry I threw the box at him and left the room. Turns out he had left over wrapping paper and thought he would use it up and wrap up his old ring box from his high school hockey ring.

—THE SLIME THAT MEN DO!!!

Just Got Married… To a Slime
—Tamara L'Ecuyer

I got married in September 1993. We didn't make any special plans for a honeymoon but thought that something would fall into place just before the wedding. We were both young and naïve. We took one week off of work and figured we'd either stay around town (we live 15 minutes from Niagara Falls) or go somewhere not too far. Well, it turns out that with a suggestion from my new husband, we ended up going to Edmonton, Alberta. **WHO DOESN'T WANT TO HONEYMOON THERE, THEY HAVE A BIG MALL.**

That is not the problem. The problem is that we drove through the U.S. in a little GMC S10 pickup truck (for two days that is) we didn't have U.S. money and no hotel or gas station wanted to take Canadian money at 11:00 at night. So, we slept in the truck bed in a bank parking lot (in Michigan) until the bank opened at 9:00 A.M. **OH, THAT'S THE PROBLEM.**

It turns out that if you don't have a bank account or know someone with one, they don't want to take Canadian money either, but after begging the teller for about 15 minutes I talked them into exchanging $60^{00} just so that we could get gas because that is all we needed. **THIS SEEMS TO BE GOING VERY WELL.**

After all that we didn't stay in a hotel to have some "newlywed privacy," no, we had to stay with one of my NEW husband's best friends who it turns out is living in a trailer that was converted from a bus. **CLASSY.** I guess I should have figured out that this was not a good start to the marriage because as you can guess, we are now divorced. **NO, SHOCKING. YOU MEAN THIS DIDN'T WORK OUT???**

I hope you get a good laugh out of this, because I still laugh at it and so do my friends. —THE SLIME THAT NEWLYWED MEN DO

Slime Told To Me... Worst Birthday Ever!!

Ok, my husband of 11 years had planned a surprise birthday party for me at our cabin for the weekend. As far as I knew, we had a very happy, very blissful marriage. And, it was a very happy birthday party, and he invited all of our friends some of whom he had flown into this place. We were all having a gay old time. *MUCH LIKE THE FLINTSTONES.*

At one point in the evening I looked at the beautiful new gold and diamond watch he had just given me. *SOUNDS LIKE A DECENT GUY, SURPRISE PARTY, BIG EXPENSIVE WATCH AND THEN...*

He'd been missing for about a half an hour. Looked at my watch again. Yes, it's been half an hour. Looked at my watch yet again and thought this is really, really strange. I better go see if I can find him. So I looked around and I end up going into one of the rooms we use as a guest room. And I couldn't open that door. Then I went to the other side and that door was still locked and I thought there's only one other way in there: through the screen. And lo and behold, what do I see when I look in there? My husband with my best girlfriend. *NOT FOR LONG.*

That's not the half of it! Well, they were going at it. Anyhow, he looks up at me with those far away eyes and says "It's not what you think Hon—it's not what you think!" I said what the heck is it then? *RESEARCH MAYBE?*

They just laid there. So I get very, very angry. And I took this gorgeous watch that the loser had given me and I ran as fast as I could to the lake and I threw it in. And all he could say was, "It's not insured! It's not insured!" Loser. Major loser.   —THE SLIME THAT MEN DO

Slime Told To Me... Slime At Birth

A lot of your slime seem to involve people who shouldn't be slipping between the sheets—it's about sex with the wrong people, that type of thing. My story is about my guy who in the heat of, uh, battle said the most bizarre thing. *BATTLE? MAYBE SHE WAS MARRIED TO BRAVEHEART.*

This is sort of a sweet bit of slime. It involves a sensitive new age guy.

You know, caring, attentive, listens, shares wants to be with his wife, and wants to be with her through everything, good and bad. *THOSE GUYS REALLY WRECK IT FOR THE REST OF US.*

Anyway I was in labor and hubby was my labor coach, encouraging me through the whole thing. It's our first baby so it's taking a long time and he's there all the way through. We've already taken the prenatal classes, we've been doing the breathing he's even read stories to the baby in my tummy and played classical music to the fetus. *OY.*

So we're at the final hour. He's doing all the things right by the book, just like a sensitive new age guy would do. So they finally wheel me into the delivery room, and it takes even more time. I'm now in real pain, like we're talking major pain. *THE KIND OF PAIN ONLY A WOMAN CAN BE IN… I FEEL YOU SISTER.*

So I'm in there and having a tough time, and all of a sudden he leans over, Mr. Sensitive, and whispered those words that every woman wants to hear… Those words were: "Honey, are you gonna be much longer? My back is killing me."

WELL SO LONG SENSITIVE MAN HELLO REGULAR SELFISH GUY…

—The Slime That Men Do

Slime and Cancer Free
—Sandy Johnson

Well have I got one for you! In January of 2004 I was diagnosed with breast cancer. As you can imagine, this rocked my stable little world. I had no idea what was to follow. I had surgery in Feb. 2004 which successfully removed the cancerous tumor. *GREAT TO HEAR.* It was shortly after this (just before my radiation treatments were starting) that my husband of 22 years announced he hadn't been happy for years and it was all my fault! *WHAT AN ASS.*

Within two months he had taken up residence with his boss's secretary and oh yeah, they had always "just been friends!" (She's a ditzy blond who incidentally left her husband just after he had open heart surgery!) ***THE TWO OF THEM ARE PERFECT FOR EACH.***

So there you go-two "slime stories in one!" The good news here is I just had my two-year check up and I am cancer free! I'm also enjoying life more than I ever could have imagined. Take care...***CANCER AND SLIME-FREE...***   —THE SLIME THAT MEN DO.

23 Years of Slime
—Mara Cole

Where to start. I could literally write all day!

I think one of my pinnacle moments came when we were out for my second son's third birthday. Hubby chose this particular day to unload all his sinful secrets on me, in the middle of the Organ Grinder no less. The name of the restaurant certainly is ironic, given the type of secrets he chose to share, and suffice it to say, my son's birthday brings mixed feelings to this day.

If that wasn't bad enough, the birth of my third son was an emergency C-section. He was born at 2:55 A.M. and by 7:00 A.M. hubby was on his way to a pre-planned business trip out of town. Thanks. Like by the third kid you don't know enough to stick around? Now, SOME men might have arranged for a nice ride home for mommy and baby... maybe even a limo. Not my guy! He had arranged NOTHING, and so, just 24 hours after the C-section, I took a cab home with my newborn, in order to look after all three kids on my own. ***SOUNDS LIKE A GREAT GUY—WHAT'S THE PROBLEM?***

This gem of a man finally left, after 23 years of marriage and three kids. He left by SENDING ME AN E-MAIL one Sunday night three years ago. Yes, I have done one better than the *Sex and the City* Post-it Note episode, I think!

Ladies, I cried for one day and one day only. Then I hired a moving truck and sent his things to his mother's… and THAT's a whole other story! —THE SLIME THAT MEN DO

Slime Times Three
—JoAnne

Listening to your show in the mornings on my drive into work has given me the courage to put into writing what I have been going through over the past two years and hopefully bring awareness to other women going through the same ordeal or maybe bring a bit of humor to the day. *THANK YOU.*

It first started off with my husband of 23 years telling me the day before my birthday that he wanted a divorce and then his cell phone rang with a girl on the other end and he left. He even had the nerve to call me the next day to wish me a Happy Birthday! *NICE GUY.* My reply to him was—Where do I send the lawyer's papers? That turned out to the best birthday present I have ever received.

Next I met a younger man who convinced me to loan him a lot of money and then he dumped me by sending me an e-mail message that he was going to go back to his wife two weeks later. I am still trying to get that money back! *GOOD LUCK WITH THAT.*

Then I met an older man who I was with for 10 months who told me that he went out on Friday nights because he wanted to be single and was looking to see if he could find someone more his type. He broke up with me by leaving me a voicemail message that he was going to marry the woman he used to live with. *ISN'T THAT SPECIAL*

Things seem to happen in threes for me so I feel my curse is over now. I feel that things can only get better now in my life. *I HOPE SO TOO NOW THAT YOU'RE FINISHED WITH…*

—THE SLIME THAT MEN DO

Slime Wrestling
—Rose Christie

Here is my story:

After 11 years of marriage my husband (ex, now, LOL) decided that the "mud wrestling" tickets he had won would make a wonderful anniversary present. Personally I think he was thinking of his own interests (haha). Being the trouper I am I did not complain and went along with this. Before going to the show we went to Turtle Jacks in Brampton where we met a male friend who was accompanying us to the show (wow what an anniversary). *SOUNDS GREAT, YOU—HIM—HIS BUDDY AND MUD WRESTLING!*

While at Turtle Jacks I informed the waitress it was our anniversary and asked her to guess where my husband was taking me. Of course her guesses were wrong. *YOU MEAN SHE DIDN'T GUESS MUD-WRESTLING.* She got the manager and they both came to our table and I told them where we were going. The manager and the waitress told my husband he was lucky I was not divorcing him (that came 1 year later.)

—THE SLIME THAT MEN DO

Special Delivery For Mr. Slime
—Leigh-Anne Kellock

I was in the delivery room in labor with our second child. My husband, leafing through a magazine and sitting back in a nice comfy rocking chair, looks up at me and asks "Is this going to take long?" *NICE.*

As I stared at him in disbelief he paused a moment then went back to reading his magazine.

After the baby was born he asked me, "Do you think the doctor will let you stay in the hospital an extra night? I really want to go to my Christmas Party!" *GREAT GUY—GREAT DAD.*

By this point I am just happy at the thought of not having to look at his face an extra night so I arrange it. But the best part of this story is the morning the baby and I are released I get a call from my "joy of a husband" to tell me that the receptionist at work left his car door open a bit last night so his battery is dead. He is going to be a bit late. After waiting for another two hours I called my mom and dad to come and pick us up.

Needless to say he has a well deserved EX in front of his title now! *HE MAY BE YOUR EX, BUT HE WILL ALWAYS QUALIFY FOR...*

—THE SLIME THAT MEN DO

Ring Around the Slime, Part 2
—Nancy

My husband has left a wound so deep, I wonder if I'll ever trust a man again.

I was married ten years and 11 months when I finally left—almost nine years ago and I haven't had more than a couple of dates since. (Trust me, I'm considered very above average in the looks and personality department, however, the majority of friends and family will not set me up or introduce me to prospective partners because THEY feel no one could measure up to ME, plus I'm considered a pretty good catch—good job and income, no children, my own house, car, VERY independent, but still quite lonely.) *MUCH LIKE MYSELF*

My ex & I traveled extensively throughout the US following the NASCAR racing circuit, visiting tracks, attending races, auctions, etc. He always dreamed of going to the Richard Petty Racing School at Charlotte Motor Speedway, so for our 10th Wedding Anniversary I secretly got him a gift certificate for the one day course (a costly $1500 U.S.) *NICE.*

Understand that when we were first engaged, I picked out my own engagement & wedding ring and choose a small (petite) diamond set, knowing it was all we could afford. For two years prior to our 10th, I started hinting about the tenth wedding anniversary diamond band that they always advertised. I walked past jewellery shops and commented on the styles and designs. I paid for our contribution to the group lottery at our place of work (yea, we worked in the same building) and always joked with co-workers that he had to save his money for my ring, in his presence. ***HMMM, I WONDER IF HE WAS GETTING THE HINT!***

So, there we were. Fancy restaurant, my nice card with the gift certificate, and he literally didn't have a THING. No card, no ring, no intention of even getting a ring. That night was the second time in my marriage that I cried. The first time was when my dog died. When I woke up the next day (being a Saturday) he wasn't home. When he returned, he THREW a jewellery bag across the room at me and said "HERE'S YOUR F——ING!!! RING, I HOPE YOU'RE HAPPY NOW." ***WHAT A DICK. YES I SAID 'DICK'!***

My marriage was over in that moment, not to mention he used my credit card to buy the ring. Eleven months later, I finally left. He never understood how selfish and slimey that was. He tried to fix things, but the damage was done, it was far too late. He hurt me more than I could ever forgive. If there was ever a slimey guy—HE'S THE ONE!!

—The Slime That Men Do

The Many Layers of Slime
—Ali

Oh where do I begin.

My ex-husband, is a SLIME (I truly am ashamed to admit I married this guy.) I was expecting our daughter at the time and I had a feeling he was having an affair. Oh no Howard, that isn't the real slime. His slime comes in layers. Anyhow, he had said he had to go away "on business" for the weekend. ***MONKEY BUSINESS.*** He said he was going to leave me the car so I could get around. How nice. Later in the day I had to go out and when I went to the car it had been ransacked. The glove box was opened and everything thrown around. CDs everywhere. I couldn't believe it. Did someone break into the car? Hmmm there were no signs of the car being broken into. The doors were still locked.

After calling the swine to tell him, he said not to worry about it and to make sure the car was working alright. (????????) *????????* OK, I thought. The car was dead! I told him I would call up a friend of ours (a mechanic). He said he would do it for me. I should go rest. The friend came later in the evening and said that the car needed a new part and that because it was so late, there was nothing he could do and that he would have to order the part which wouldn't come in until Monday, so I may as well wait until the swine got back. Howard are you seeing the layers? *TO BE HONEST I'M A LITTLE CONFUSED. HELP.*

Here is the punchline: when the swine got back he went to look at the car and called me a stupid idiot because all I had to do was switch off the interior light which had drained the battery. That swine left the light on all night to drain the battery, knew the car wouldn't work, called his friend to tell me some crap and miraculously discovered the little light switch on top of the car was in the on position. Well Howard, there it is. Slime in layers. Please let me know if you need anymore slimey stories for your book. If this wasn't what you had in mind and wanted something slimier (is that even a word?) let me know. I have tons. *I'M NOT SURE WHAT THE HELL THIS WAS ALL ABOUT…BUT I APPRECIATE THE STORY OF…*

—THE SLIME THAT MEN DO (I THINK????)

Slime Across The Ocean
—Angie

Here is my slime that men do story.

My then-husband and I had planned a trip to England after I finished my last semester of college. As we were sitting waiting to board the plane he informed me that he had been thinking of leaving me and that I had the two weeks we were in England to prove myself to him. *NICE.* Of course at this point I wanted to try and save my marriage so I spent the next week trying to figure out what I had done wrong and trying to make things right. Two days before we were scheduled to fly home I woke up in the morning to find him standing at the bedroom door staring at me. He told me to go back to sleep so I did, I just figured he was going for his morning run like he had been doing the whole time we were there. When I did wake up I found that he was gone. As in he had flown home. **NO WAY** He had taken his knapsack but left the rest of his luggage and went to the corner and taken a cab to the airport, bought himself a new ticket and flown home. He did leave a note that simply said "it's not enough to love, you must be in love." **HOW BOTH PROFOUND AND SLIMEY.** To add insult to injury, we had taken his car to the airport so I had to call my parents to come pick me up when I landed as I had no way to get home.

Some say hindsight is twenty twenty. Looking back I now realize that he had been cheating on me during our marriage and he actually had the balls to cheat on me while we were in England together and this was his way of getting out of the marriage. I'd say it was a little overboard. **I'D AGREE, NOT ONLY OVERBOARD BUT MORE OF...**

—THE SLIME THAT MEN DO

Long, Painful, Slime Story — But Worth It
—Jane
(the names have been changed to protect the innocent!)

My slime story probably should fall under the category of "What REALLY Stupid Things Women Put Up With In the Name of Love," but, I guess it will work in the slime category too. **TOO LONG.**

In my opinion, my first husband wins the award for the slimiest character that ever crossed my path—unfortunately it took me 8 years to realize it and get out—here are just some of the examples of what I put up with.

When we were engaged he (let's call him DICK, just for fun), **DICK...YOU'RE RIGHT, THAT WAS FUN. TEE HEE** was stationed in

Germany. We wrote to each other frequently for several months. In one of those many love letters he asked me "how I would react if I knew that he had a child with another woman?" **WHAT??** Well, after several weeks of wondering, DICK told me that it was all a test, or joke, shall we say, to see how I would react and that it really wasn't true. **OH THAT'S SOME FREAKING HILARIOUS JOKE, DICK.**

Our "very special" wedding night consisted of dinner at Burger King and a hotel 15 minutes from home. Our "well thought out and romantic" (HAH!) honeymoon consisted of a three-hour drive down the highway (until we got tired of driving) and then a hotel for three days of room service (which was the most fun) and the usual endless "rolling in the hay." **TOO BAD THEY DIDN'T HAVE BEDS.** But, during the first night, in the heat of the moment, DICK called out, "OH CONNIE!" Well, that is NOT my name! He made up some lame excuse and laughed it off. **STRANGE SENSE OF HUMOUR.**

Shortly after we were married, we went out to a bar in our home-town to socialize with old friends. DICK spent the whole evening at the bar with his old girlfriend, and ignored me. When I questioned him later about it, DICK said "I had to make sure I still have "it," just in case we ever get divorced." **THAT'S JUST ABOUT THE STRANGEST B.S. I'VE EVER HEARD.**

When I had our daughter, a year later, we lived about eight hours from any friends or family. My "slime ball" husband only showed up at the hospital for a few minutes each day to visit. The day I got out of the hospital, after having my beautiful daughter, my stupid, uncaring husband made me sit in the car (OUCH!!!) for the eight-hour drive to our hometown, where DICK had the urge to go out and celebrate the birth of his child with his brothers and friends and leave me home with our new baby. **NOW HE'S FATHER OF THE YEAR!**

Countless times DICK would, "go out for cigarettes" and not return for 6–12 hours, at which time he would stagger into my parent's house, where we stayed while home visiting and act like a total drunken fool. **CIGARETTES GET YOU DRUNK?**

He loved attention from any and all women, for a boost to his ego and had no problem flirting in front of me. But, if any guy even so much as looked my way, DICK would stick his chest out, grab onto me and say to the person, "What the "F" are you looking at?" I was so embarrassed by his behaviour that I started to go out without him just to be alone have fun without that stress. *I'M GUESSING YOU GUYS AREN'T STILL MARRIED???*

So, fast forward to the present (19 years after my hellish marriage ended) DICK has been married three times now! Each marriage worse than the one before. He and his current wife are very well known for their bar room brawls and drunken behaviour. *THEY SOUND LIKE FUN.*

I, thankfully, am remarried to the kindest, most wonderful man that ever lived and have a wonderful life, THANK YOU GOD! And the thing that I am most thankful for is that I never have to lay an eye on my slime-ball EX-Husband again! AMEN!!! *RIGHT ON SISTAH.*

I know that this was kind of lengthy, but it sure does make a girl appreciate what she has now and it also may help women in similar relationships realize that all is not lost! Life changes all of the time, especially when you least expect it!

—The Slime That "Dicks" Do

Bachelor Party Slime
—Tricia Colibaba

Here is a story that I now find humor in as the years have gone by.

My soon-to-be husband and I lived together shortly before our marriage in 1994. His friends had taken him out for a night on the town just prior to our wedding. I had gone out to get some things done for the wedding while my fiancé and his best buddies were out doing things that I would rather not have too much knowledge of. *TRUST ME YOU DON'T WANT TO KNOW.* I showed up at our apartment in the wee hours of the morning only to find Doug (my fiancé) lying passed out on our living room floor with all of his buddies still partying. Out of concern for my future husband, I walked over to make sure that he was okay. He was still breathing, but totally out cold. *SOUNDS LIKE HUBBY-TO-BE HAD FUN.* Upon further inspection, I noticed that he had lipstick in the shape of lips imprinted on his cheek!! I asked his best friend where they had been. Colin said that Doug had been enjoying himself at a strip joint. Of course the boys all had a good laugh at watching the future bride getting angry about the evidence that had been left on the cheek. I kicked the guys out and then fetched a Kleenex. I pressed the tissue over the lipstick on Doug's cheek and got a perfect impression of the lips to show him when he came-to. *VERY CSI OF YOU!*

Doug had no idea where the lipstick had come from when confronted the next morning. After asking the best friend about the big night out, we finally found out that the boys thought that it would be funny to have Colin put on some of my lipstick and plant a big wet one on Doug while he was passed out. *HYSTERICAL, RIGHT?* The highlight of the night was waiting for me to come home and see my reaction. This truly was slimey. We are now happily married with three lovely children. Yes, Doug is still friends with Colin. He still has some slimey outbursts, but when they are not directed at you, he really is a funny guy. *OH I'LL BET HE'S A REAL SCREAM...*   —THE SLIME THAT MEN DO

To Catch A Slime
—Carolyn

At least I can laugh about it now. Flash back to 1995.

I thought that my husband at the time was fooling around on me. With two small children and a full time job to manage, I think that he thought I was to busy to find out. But a woman always knows. *CUE THE SCARY "A WOMEN ALWAYS KNOWS" MUSIC...*

Anyway, being the small time PI that I was, I had been checking his pockets and such and on the evening of February 13th I found a key for the local motel in his coat pocket. *YOU DIDN'T HAVE TO DO MUCH INVESTIGATION TO START THE SLIME BALL ROLLING...*

I didn't say anything to him, but come the next morning after he left for 'work' I phoned the motel and they confirmed that indeed, he had checked in. I told the woman on the phone that I was his wife and was meeting him there for a

Valentines Day tryst and needed the room number. *THE PLOT THICKENS.* She gave it to me!

I dropped the kids off at daycare and drove to the motel. Sure enough, both his car and the car of his 25-year-old employee was there. *OOPSY.*

I went to the door and listened. Did you know you can hear everything through the door of a motel room? *UH, NO, WHY WHAT HAVE YOU HEARD? OH, YOU WEREN'T ASKING ME... I KNEW THAT.*

I knocked on the door and when he said "Yes, can help you?" I said, "Room service" Keeping in mind that there is no room service in a motel like this, he answered "I didn't order room service" I then proceeded to tell him that I knew he was in there with so and so and that I was off to tell her parents who and what she was doing!!! *DUDE WAS SO BUSTED.*

I went to the car and sure enough he ran out shortly thereafter and got into my car. Obviously I was upset and proceeded to scream at him telling him that that was going to be the most expensive f**k he ever had! Instead of apologizing or begging forgiveness, he tells me calmly "I only met her so that I could tell her it was over" *OH YEAH THAT'S THE EXPLANTATION YOU WERE LOOKING FOR...LIKE YOU'D GO "OH WELL THAT'S OKAY THEN, LET'S GO FOR A DRINK!"*

Right! You're in a hotel room on Valentines Day; you meet your girlfriend to tell her it was over—give me a break! Anyway, fast forward 11 years later and I am now divorced from him and am in love with a wonderful man who treats me like a princess and I have never been so happy in my entire life. *YOU MEAN HE DOESN'T SCREW AROUND WITH HIS MISTRESS ON VALENTINES DAY?*

—THE SLIME THAT MEN DO

You Think This Stuff Only Happens in the Movies...
—Anon. by request, you'll see why

I was slated to be married on May 19, 2001. This day was the culmination of a six-year relationship that had seen it's ups and downs, but I thought was always bountiful with love. We had a son in 1998, and I was excited about the fact that we would finally be a family. Unfortunately, in the week leading up to the wedding, our son came down with the chicken pox and therefore would not be able to attend the ceremony. Although we lived in Toronto, we were getting married in my hometown of Chatham, ON. The wedding was going to be a small affair, 50 people, just close friends and families. All the replies had been received and everyone confirmed attendance, with the exception of one person from my side, and one person from his side. **WHY DOES THAT SOUND OMINOUS?**

On the day of the wedding rehearsal my then–fiancé was fielding calls throughout the afternoon, from his groomsmen who "advised" that they were having challenges making it to Chatham in time for the rehearsal as childcare arrangements for one of the groomsmen had fallen through. There were only two groomsmen and they were coming together. I was quite upset but thought there's nothing I can do about it, so we went through with the rehearsal. We had a barbecue afterwards at my sister's house, with my immediate family and some very close friends. My fiancé continued to take calls from his "groomsmen" who then advised they would not be there until first thing in the morning. Given the flaky character of his groomsmen I wasn't surprised by the string of events. I was a little nervous, but the excitement of the next day overshadowed this. **OKAY SO FAR, FLAKY GROOMSMEN AND ALL.**

My former fiancé was staying at my sister and brother-in-law's until the wedding. On my wedding day, my mom, sister and I set out early to get our hair and make-up done. The wedding was at 4 P.M. We were finished our hair and make-up by about 10:30 A.M. My sister called to speak with her husband, and I asked to speak with my fiancé.

Apparently, he had gone out to play a round of golf with the "grooms-men" and wasn't back yet. I was getting a little concerned as the cars needed to be decorated with flowers. Nevertheless, my sister dropped me off at our parents house, and went back to her house to get dressed for the wedding. My sister returned to my parents house just after 1 P.M., dressed in her brides-maid outfit. She then broke the news to me and my parents that my fiancé hadn't returned and she didn't know where he was. *NOW IT'S GETTING NOT GOOD.*

We were all beside ourselves at the time wondering what had happened. My mom took off to the hotel, to see if she could find the groomsmen. Lo and behold, they had not checked into the hotel. My mom then went to tell the priest that the groom had gone A-Wall. *AWOL, BUT I THINK WE GET IT.* The poor priest didn't know what to do, as this had never happened before. He sought counsel from another priest in town who told him that it was too late to stop the wedding, and to open the doors of the church to greet the guests. At about 2:30 P.M., I called my former fiancé's house. A lady picked up the phone, and I asked if my fiancé was there. She replied he wasn't, and that he wouldn't be back until Sunday as he was on a business trip to the U.S. When I heard that response, I asked who she was, and she replied "his wife." Needless to say, I lost it! I came to learn that he had been married since 1997 and had another son, who was eight months old at the time! *YOU-ARE-KIDDING??? (STUNNED LOOKS ON EVERY-ONE'S FACES)*

The bottom line was he was leading a double life! She was shocked to learn that we were to be getting married that day and that we had a son almost 3-years-old (at that time). My father, sister, best friend and the priest had to announce to a church full of my family and friends that there would not be a wedding. My brother-in-law eventually found my car at the train station with a note from my former fiancé advising he had contacted all of his guests that the wedding was called off and that he couldn't marry me, and hopped a train to Chicago. I know this seems 'way out there' but this is the God's truth as to what happened to me five years ago. If that's not a slimey thing for a man to do, I don't know what is. *IT IS, SLIMEY AND COWARDLY...THE SLIME THAT ONLY A VERY FEW (THANKFUL) MEN DO.*

Uh, I Think This Slime Wants Me To Take A Survey...
—Lyndsay

OK here is a true slime ball!

My story begins when my "other half" Rick, our $1^1/_2$-year old son and I moved from BC back to Toronto where most of our family resides. Being a single income family at the time we didn't have much money, but my grandmother had passed away I had used some of my inheritance to pay for the flight and to rent a new apartment. My 'other half' quickly found a night job as a telemarketer (I should have known at that point!) *OOOH YEAH, TELEMARKETERS CAN BE VERY SLIMEY...* He soon started returning from work with stories of his day, many featuring his new co-worker Courtney. I had a twinge of feminine intuition but ignored it (stupid, stupid me). I met Court (as she had become) once, when my son and I went to meet Rick for dinner. *NICK-NAMES MEAN SOMETHING'S GOING ON...* I was forced to introduce myself when Rick didn't, she never said hi to me just told Rick how much our son looked like him which is really funny because I could have cloned this child, we look identical. At this point seeing the inter-action between the two of them loud alarms started ringing in my head. When we had a moment alone I asked him if there was anything to be concerned about. I was given a long speech about how he loved me and only me and there was nothing to worry about. *OF COURSE THAT'S ALL BS RIGHT?*

About a month after our return to Toronto, Rick asked me to go to my parents for a while because he needed time to think things through (keep in mind he is "thinking things through" in the apartment I paid for!) He gave me a speech about how we are still a couple, he loves me and is interested in no one else but needs some time for himself. *HE'S REALLY JUST LOOKING TO SPEND SOME TIME WITH "COURT!"*

One day follows another fairly quickly and we hear very little from Rick but when I do speak to him its the same story, he loves and misses us. Then one day I hear from the landlord he is looking for rent and

Rick won't pay. Well I may have been stupid (I freely admit this) but not even I am that stupid to pay rent for a place I'm no living in, so feeling pretty ticked off I arrange a day to pick up my son's and my possessions. I asked Rick to please be there so that we might be able to talk and work this out and he agreed. When I arrived, Rick was just leaving, saying he had a great job interview that he cannot pass up. I know he's lying and asked him to stay but he refused, saying he loves me and we will talk when he returned. As I am packing I notice that he has added a new name to our autodial: "Court." I hit the button. "Hi," I say to Courtney "This is Jen, Rick's sister, I just stopped by his house for a visit and he's not home. Do you know where he is?" "Sure" she answers "he's on his way here. We are going to look at apartments together." *OOPS.* My heart stopped but knowing maybe this is nothing I steady my voice and say "Oh I hate to be nosey but are you moving in as roommates or are you a couple?" "We're a couple but don't tell his ex she doesn't know yet." *SHE DOES NOW!!! BUSTED.*

Fuming I ask her to tell him to give me a call at his house when he arrives.

Needless to say, when he called our conversation was not pretty. After five years I had to learn that we were not together from his new girlfriend and he wasn't planning on telling me. *NICE, CLASSY TOUCH...*
—The Slime That Men Do

Slime Surprise!!!
—Anon.

My husband was throwing a surprise birthday party for me. He invited twenty of our closest friends, put up balloons, had the event catered, and had everyone dress up. Everyone was wearing their suits. *FANCY-LIKE.* Yeah, and I had bought myself a beautiful new dress, had my hair done, and he was really happy that I looked so pretty. I should tell you my husband and I had been married seven years. *OKAY.* I thought everything was going great. We had no problems, we agreed about money, we had no arguments. I walked through the door and everyone shouted "Surprise!" And it was really fun. And then he decided to do a toast at about twelve o'clock. *NICE, A BIRTHDAY TOAST.*

You know, I had tears in my eyes because it was so nice that somebody had done this for me, and I was standing there and everyone was holding their glasses. He made this wonderful toast to his wife, how wonderful I was and how good I was, how sexy and beautiful. And then he said "I would like a divorce." And he handed me *(EVERYONE'S' HEAD SHAKES) WHAT????* divorce papers. *HAPPY FREAKING BIRTHDAY!!* He felt that he couldn't do it if he was by himself, that he would chicken out. He wanted to have the strength of a party atmosphere, toss a few back and he figured that would give him the nerve to do it. But I was crushed and my friends were horrified. Needless to say it was my worst birthday ever. *NO KIDDING...THE SLIME THAT SPINELESS GUYS DO*

Me Slime You Jane
—Nadine

Okay, there's a friend of ours, her name is Debbie, she was supposed to be getting married last year. So we threw a wedding shower for her. She'd known the guy for approximately a year, and he told her he was a businessman or a salesman or something. *SOUNDS FINE SO FAR.* Yes, and he was really nice, really good, took her out, bought her flowers, all the usual. Anyway, we decided the shower should have a male stripper. *OF COURSE.* Right, so the shower was going great, everybody was having a good time, all the girls were laughing and drinking. The doorbell rings and we think okay, this has got to be him, this is our male stripper. We'd asked for a Tarzan kind of person, so he could pick her up throw her over her shoulder and run away with her. *WHO DOESN'T WANT TARZAN SHOWING UP AT YOUR HOUSE?* Little did we know it was her fiancé. *NO WAY.* We hired some random guy out of the book and it turns out to be her fiancé? Nobody knew that he was a male stripper, including Debbie. Apparently she had never seen his loin-cloth before? *I'M SURE SHE'D SEEN HIS VINE!* So, he walks in the door and poor Debbie, there's her fiancé. *SO WHAT HAPPENS?* Well. Let's just put it this way. She was just so hurt and embarrassed plus the obvious mistrust, they never ended up getting married.

TURNS OUT TARZAN WAS A REAL CHEETAH!!! THE SLIME THAT MEN IN LOINCLOTHS DO

Surviving Slime And More
—D. Bradley

I have waited three long years to tell this story, it is cathartic for me and I thank you, no, *commend* you for allowing people to tell their stories. As a breast cancer survivor thank you. *YOU'RE WELCOME, THANK YOU.*

My guy and I had a house, we'd been together 12 years and engaged for six. My chemotherapy had finished and radiation had just completed but I was receiving no money as all my benefits had run out. I'm a nurse and I was to return to work for four-hour shifts a few days a week to gain my strength back. My fiancé decided he had had enough. He wasn't really all that supportive during my sick time—emotionally absent most of the time—and told my 18-year-old daughter (who decided not to go to college to help out with bills) that he loved her but couldn't see growing old with me, *WOW, YOU WEREN'T KIDDING WHEN YOU SAID NO-SUPPORTIVE.*

This man had been her stepfather for years and she was devastated and of course called me at work. This man was not even man enough to talk to me but told his friends that we talked for hours and decided to end the relationship. This wasn't true. He said "let her see how it feels to pay all the bills." Don't forget I was trying to get my health back, going through chemically induced menopause so didn't know if I was coming or going. The phone got cut off, the cable, the internet, the gas and all the while he harassed me to leave the house we both owned. I eventually did for my own sanity and safety. He put the house up for sale without my knowledge. *IT JUST GETS BETTER AND BETTER WITH THIS ASS.* He tormented me, he then let a production company use the house for a movie, and he was upset I found out he was getting paid for that. *HOLY CRAP!* I lost my breast, my hair, my self-esteem my home, my precious dog, everything! I have lived like a fugitive for three years hiding from this man, the man who once said I was his world and he would take a bullet for me. WELL KEITH HERE IS YOUR BULLET.

Thanks for this. D.Bradley breast cancer survivor of four years and going strong. *KEEP GOING STRONG D. AND AS FOR YOUR DUDE... I WOULDN'T WASTE A SLIME THAT MEN DO ON HIM... HE DOESN'T EVEN DESERVE THAT.*

Slime With A Twist!
—Stephen

Let me give a bit of background to set this up. My son was born six years ago. He had numerous health issues and we thought he was not going to survive. Everyday I was at work I would get phone calls from the hospital to say that I better leave work and get over there as soon as possible. When we brought Michael home from the hospital, he was put on a breathing machine for about six months then at that time he needed to have surgery on his throat. Let me state that Michael, my son, is now six and is as healthy as any child can be. *GREAT TO HEAR.*

While my son was still undergoing treatment for various illnesses my partner decided that being home all the time was not desired. I was left to take care of our son alone. My partner would stay out all night, coming home at 2 or 3 A.M. with no explanation as to where or what she had been doing. *THAT'S NOT RIGHT.* Then, on my birthday, when our son was just past a year old, my birthday gift from my partner was to tell me that they had been seeing someone else for the past 4 months and is now leaving us for this other person. *WOW.* The twist to this story is that it was my *wife* who cheated and left me alone to raise our child. I left my job of 11 years as a law clerk to take care of him. I have raised him on my own for the past $5^1/_2$ years. By the way, I have sole custody now and I am back to work. I thought I would share this with you so that there is at least one story where you can say, The Slime That Women Do! *I ABSOLUTELY WILL...*

—THE SLIME THAT WOMEN DO.

Diseased By a Slime
—BL from Oshawa

My common-law husband of thirteen years came home with a transmittable disease. He didn't know what it was at that time and was kind of freaking out so he showed me and asked me what I thought it was, (it was scabies which can only be transmitted skin to skin). *THAT DOESN'T SOUND LIKE FUN.* I had my suspicions (I must be stupid to have been with such a loser but I'm not that stupid) and advised him that he should go immediately to the clinic to see a doctor which he did. *OKAY.* When he returned, he told me what the doctor had told him and said he had gotten 'it' from the dirt in the yard as he was building a deck at the side of the house. *YES, DIRT, UH THAT'S RIGHT I GOT SCABIES FROM DIRT???* When I vocalized my disbelief, he got mad at me and stormed off. He proceeded over the next few days to 'try' and convince me of his 'doctor's' diagnoses, which I was still calling him on.

After a few days when he realized that I didn't believe him, he changed his story. This one is even better, he blamed his 'problem' on my fifteen year old son saying that 'he' brought it into the house and had transferred it to the sofa where it was transferred to my charming 'EX.' *YEAH, THE SOFA, THAT'S RIGHT THE SOFA GOT SCABIES FROM YOUR SON AND NOW I HAVE IT???*

So not only did he cheat, he also lied and he was slimey enough to try and pass the blame on to a child! SLIME!!!!!!!!

That was three years ago and he is still with the charmer who gave it to him LOL! *WAIT A MINUTE, YOU MEAN HE DIDN'T GET THE SCABIES FROM THE SOFA OR THE DECK DIRT!!!*   —THE SLIME THAT MEN DO

Have your own **MARRIED SLIME** story?

E-mail your story to **slime@humblehoward.com** and it could be included in our next book, *The Slime That Men Do 2!*

Here, make some notes, it could be therapeutic:

_____

_____

_____

_____

_____

_____

_____

_____

_____

_____

_____

_____

_____

_____

_____

_____

_____

STUPID CUPID

Happy Valentines Day From Fred Fartstone
—Barb White

My ex-husband had a very bad habit of going out with the boys on Friday nights and not coming home until noon on Saturday, extremely hung-over, which made him pretty useless for the whole day. ***THIS EXPLAINS THE EX.***

This particular Valentines Day fell on a Saturday and we had made plans to spend the entire day together. With this in mind, I had presumed that he was going to forgo his usual Friday night with the boys and stay at home that evening.

Well, come the Friday evening as I patiently waited for him to come home with dinner ready, I soon realized that he had no intention of coming home and that it was going to be the usual Friday evening.

With the plans we had made for the Saturday, we had to make a very early start, and had a babysitter arranged for 7:30 A.M. When he had not come home by 7:00 A.M. ***OOPS.*** I called the babysitter and cancelled. I waited for him to call and advise when he would be coming home, but never received one. This was before the days of cell phones, so I was unable to reach him. He finally showed up around 10 A.M. bearing a gift in a plastic bag, with no apology for ruining our plans for the day. ***AT LEAST HE HAD A GIFT!*** I threw the gift back at him and told him where to stick it. He then opened it to show me what he had bought me. It was a sweatshirt with Dino the dinosaur (Flintstones) lying on his back in a daze, paws in the air with the logo reading "Fred Fartstone U" with the motto "Yabba Dabba Pew." ***WHAT GIRL WOULDN'T WANT THAT?***

Needless to say, it was the absolute worst Valentine's Day I have ever experienced and will probably never forget.   —The Slime Men Do

Quick and to the Slime
—Colleen Thornton

This story is not about me but my cousin.

My cousin told his girlfriend to get dressed up "really nice" for Valentine's Day because he was taking her to a "really special" place for dinner. He bought a $9²² Valentine's Day special bouquet of one dozen roses, gave half to his mother and gave the other half to his girlfriend when he picked her up for dinner. She had bought a new dress and shoes to wear out for the special dinner that night and was quite excited about being taken to a fancy restaurant, only to discover that his "special dinner" was a meal at the local Legion along with a bunch of drunken war veterans! **WELL THEN...**

—THE SLIME THAT LEGIONNAIRES DO?

Not One Good V-day, Seriously
Shali

Until recently I was dating a guy on and off for six years. You'd think that within the six years there would have been at least one good Valentine's Day. There wasn't. **PERHAPS YOU WOULD CARE TO LIST THEM? YES.**

1st Valentine's Together: He broke up with me for the first time after seven months of dating. **NICE.**

2nd Valentine's Together: We made it through dinner, for which I had made the reservations, but after, when we were on our way to a movie, he got called into work. I had bought him a nice gift and he bought me a card. The card he bought while we were at the mall where the restaurant was—he told me before dinner to walk around the mall for about ten minutes because he "had to go and do something." I got the card a week later after he got around to signing it. *CLASSY.*

3rd Valentine's Together: He came to visit me at school and I had bought him a really nice gift, he said he bought me a gift but "left it at home." But he lied, there was no gift. *HAPPY HAPPY.*

4th Valentine's Together: I had plans for a nice dinner at a nice place where there was a bit of a dress code. He showed up at my place wearing jeans. I was disappointed because I would have liked him to have at least dressed up a bit since he never did for our dates. So I asked him to go to the mall and buy at least a pair of khakis. This of course led to a fight which ruined the rest of the night. *HOW DID YOU LAST THIS LONG?*

Our last Valentine's Day Together: He said he was going to plan the evening and make it special since we'd never had a nice Valentine's Day. He of course didn't arrange anything. But knowing his track record, I'd already made reservations somewhere. I get to his place the night we're supposed to go out and he's lying on the couch saying he was up really late last night and he's tired. So we watched about an hour of the Sci Fi channel with his roommate, then at 9 he said he was going to bed so I told him I was just going to go home. I cried the whole hour drive home. *AW COME ON, SCI-FI WITH HIM AND HIS ROOMIE, THAT SCREAMS ROMANCE!*

Even the way he broke up with me was awful. I woke up one morning to see a text message on my phone from him. I figured it was some cute "good morning" message. Instead it's a text message saying that he cheated on me and it's over. Of all the horrible ways to break up with someone, I think a text message is the most inconsiderate. I'll just leave it at that, I won't even go into the pathetic reason he gave me for how it happened...*I'M GUESSING HE AND HIS SCI-FI BUDDY HAD SOME KIND OF WEIRD STAR TREK/BROKEBACK MOUNTAIN THING GOING ON...*

—THE SLIME THAT MEN DO

Cookies From A Slime
—Diana Tassopoulos

I was with my ex for almost 3 years. I'll start by saying, we broke up on Valentines Day *NICE.*

He had asked me to take a day off work and stay home to wait for a delivery package from him. He also told me he made lunch reservations at a fine dining restaurant. So I was all excited that morning. *SOUNDS FINE, BUT I'M GUESSING IT DOESN'T QUITE WORK OUT!!!*

Late morning, The Package arrived... I opened up a flat giant box which contained a giant cookie. *COOKIES ARE YUMMY.* The cookie looked sooo yummy except for the wonderful message on it. The cookie read: "My Darling Sandra, I miss you so, enjoy my sweet and make room for more."

SOUNDS FINE TO ME...

My name is Diana.

AWWWW, NOT SO FINE

The card included a certificate for dinner reservations! *NO WAY.*

So I called him and asked him to come over and that I was ready to go eat. He came inside and I had the cookie box open and after he read it, he said the company sent over the wrong cookie BUT I informed him that I called them and told them the situation and they told me how the same guy sent out two cookies for V-day—he had given them the wrong addresses *WOW.*

To make a long story short, he'd been cheating on me for a year! Isn't that wonderful? *NOT REALLY...*

—THE SLIME THAT MEN DO

"Worst Valentines Ever"
—Emily Cox

My Valentine's disaster story starts in the morning of February 14th, 2002.

Actually, it is more than a disaster, it would be more appropriately named the Worst Valentine's Day EVER.

My family and I received a phone call in the morning, it was one of our very close family friends whose birthday happens to be Valentine's Day. We were wishing her a happy birthday but she interrupted to say she had bad news, another of our family friends died of breast cancer earlier on in the morning. Shocked and upset, I called my boyfriend and told him I wasn't in the mood to go out and do anything huge, but would prefer to have him there with me and watch a movie. **SOUNDS REASONABLE.**

An hour before he was supposed to meet me, he called to say he's bailing on me. I was already upset and said "you're ditching your girl-friend on Valentine's Day?" and tried to justify it by telling me that he's spending it with one of his best friends (a girl) 'cause she was having a "bad day," but one of his friends was going to take me to dinner. **I'M A LITTLE LOST, HE WAS GOING TO SPEND VALENTINE'S DAY WITH ANOTHER GIRL? DIDN'T HE HEAR THAT YOU HAD HEARD SOME BAD NEWS...**

Completely pissed off that my boyfriend was spending Valentine's with another girl because she was having a bad day when my family friend died, I hung up on him. **OKAY I'M UP TO SPEED NOW!**

An hour later, his best friend shows up at my door. **STILL HAVING A LITTLE TROUBLE WITH HIS BEST FRIEND TAKING YOU OUT INSTEAD OF HIM.** My boyfriend had told him what happened and told him that I was being a "bitch" and "jealous." His best friend still took me out for dinner but "forgot his wallet" so I ended up paying a fortune for dinner. **COURSE YOU PAID, IT WOULDN'T BE THE WORST V-DAY EVER IF YOU DIDN'T!** I told him I wanted to go home, but he said that we had to go pick up his sister. So, an hour and a half later, I get home, miserable and angry. I called my boyfriend and he picks up, and I hear the chick in the background kissing him and giggling. I say that she must be having a terrible day, and he says they'd been drinking a little and that we'll talk about it later. *RIGHT.*

I call the friend who just dropped me off and asked if The Boyfriend has been cheating on me, well, my guess is you know where this is going. *I DO......*

So, I call my boyfriend back and he starts getting mad at me, so I tell him that he's an a-hole for cheating and that that was the worst thing anyone can do, and that we were done. Needless to say, he called me the next day, and apologized and begged for forgiveness, and I hung up on him and told him I never wanted to see him again.

In summary, my Valentines disaster started with a death, continued with me footing the bill for a dinner with someone I barely knew, and ended up with a cheating boyfriend and a breakup. *I THINK YOU SUMMED THAT UP NICELY, 'CEPT FOR ONE THING...*

—THE SLIME THAT MEN DO!!!!

Slime Forgot More Than Just Valentines Day
—Michelle Mester

Hi Howard. *HI MICHELLE!* Here's my story: *OKAY.*

I had been dating this guy for a couple of months when Valentine's Day rolled around. I was completely smitten with him so I made him a mixed tape (it was the early '90s, pre-MP3s or burned CDs!) *I REMEMBER THOSE* of the most romantic, lovey-dovey songs I liked. I also hand-made a wooden box and inside it I put an antique skeleton key with a note saying, "you touched my soul and now I give you the key to my heart" WOW Total cheese, I know. But I was young, dumb and totally head-over-heels. *WE'VE ALL BEEN THERE.*

Valentine's Day night he comes over. I knew things were off to a bad start when he showed up empty handed. *OOPSY.* I asked him if he would like his gift and he said, "A gift? Why did you get me a gift?" I replied, "Because it's Valentine's Day!" DUH! ***DOUBLE DUH!!***

His answer? "Oh. I totally forgot." ***BAD ANSWER.*** So I decided to let that slide and give him his gift anyway. First he opened the mixed tape and proceeded to tell me that he doesn't have a tape player. Then when he opened the box and read the note on the key he said, "I don't get it." ***COME ON.*** I had to explain to him what the key to my heart was! After that he told me that he has made plans with one of his friends and he has to go. He promptly left and I never ever heard from again. He wouldn't return my phone calls, he was never home when I went by. He just fell off the face of the earth and I never saw him again. I was devastated for quite some time. The worst part was that I never got an explanation or even a proper break-up. He just disappeared. So somewhere out in the world there is a jerk who has the key to my heart and I want it back!!! And that's my story. ***THE SLIME THAT GUYS WHO ARE TOO BIG A SUCK TO BREAK UP WITH SOMEONE FACE TO FACE AFTER THEY GAVE THEM THE KEY TO THEIR HEARTS, DO.***

Monsieur Pilot Du Slime
—Karen Johnson

I had been dating this "gentleman" for about three or four months and he suggested we go to Montreal for the Valentine's Day weekend to visit his "relatives." I was so excited to see Montreal and be with someone who spoke French and knew the city really well. ***BON BON***

We head out in his brand new Saab, all ready for a glorious three-day weekend. ***BIBLIOTHEQUE!*** Once we get into Montreal, he pulls up to a well-known hotel and says we are staying there for the Thursday, Friday and Saturday nights. So, I piled all of our stuff out of the car and hauled it into the hotel while he walked ahead of me! ***QUELLE HOLE DU ARSE.*** My "boyfriend" begin speaking in French to the desk attendant. I just smiled a lot, since I am totally clueless about anything in the French language. ***MOI AUSSI.*** His tone of voice became very argumentative and he started pounding the front desk. *TETE DU PEE PEE!* I could tell something was wrong, but I just kept smiling. He turned to me and said that we couldn't stay there, because the hotel was all booked, months in advance, because of a gynecological physicians conference. *LE DOCTOUR DU CHAT.* He never even made reservations! I was stunned!

Anyway, he said "Don't worry about it, I do this all the time, they always keep a couple of rooms open for emergencies, and you can usually get a really good deal on them." *EXCUSE MOI MONSIEUR GRAND SHOT!*

After about 15 minutes of negotiation, the front desk clerk called a bell-boy to take our luggage upstairs! I was thrilled. He did it! Little did I know that they put us in an upstairs conference room with a pull-out couch! He was so proud that he had negotiated a really good deal on a conference room! Then, to make matters worse, his "family" consisted only of his sister and brother, who he finally admitted to me that he really didn't care very much, he just wanted an excuse to go to Montreal. So we sat in total silence, at dinner, with his family staring at us like "What the hell are you doing here?" I soon found out that they didn't think much of him, either! *LES GROSS TWIT.*

After one final exhausting night on a pull-out couch we headed back to Toronto. *OH LA LA, CEST BON WEEKEND.* Now here's the clincher!!! A few days later, he called me to let me know that my "half" of our holiday to Montreal was $600! To say the least I dumped his ass! *SANS DOUBT...* —LES SLIME DUS HOMME, UH... DO.

Slime Too Sexy For My Current Chick...
—Amanda Loughlin-Lihou

It was 1998. I was madly in love. Dave and I had been going strong for four months. We were inseparable. To prove how hot I thought my sweetheart was, I entered him in a "Hot Valentine Contest" run by the *Toronto Sun*. In great detail I extolled the romantic, wonderful, sexy virtues of my love-god. I did not hold back. It was steamy. I believe I actually used the words "made me quiver." *WOW, QUIVER, I SOME-TIMES MAKE MY WIFE SHIVER, BUT ONLY WHEN I'VE LEFT THE WINDOW OPEN.*

To my surprise, he was a runner up!

In the newspaper in a dashing tuxedo was my honey, my handsome 40ish boyfriend for all the world to see. And they did.

At least 10 of his old girlfriends called him up, gushing all over and asking him out. *OF COURSE DUDE HAS 10 OLD GIRLFRIENDS, HE MAKES WOMEN QUIVER.* One ex was someone he had dated when he was 19! Long story short, he hooked up with an ex and they moved in together four months later, *OOPS* Me and my bright idea.

P.S. In 2002, on Valentines Day, my new husband proposed and we are happily married. And I won't be entering him in any contests.

—THE SLIME THAT HOT GUYS WITH LOTS OF EXS DO!!

A Crush On Prince Sliming
—Cheryl Sue

About 10 years ago when I was in second year university, I had a huge crush on this guy who lived on my floor in residence. I thought he was the most beautiful person I had seen walk the earth and would have done anything just to be with him. *MY WIFE FEELS THAT WAY ABOUT ME...OKAY EVERYBODY STOP GAGGING.*

I kept my identity secret until Hallowe'en Candy-grams were handed out in residence. When he found out who sent it to him, he seemed pretty much into me also. *COOL.* So we hung out for a few months and I really thought it could go somewhere. I should have seen the signs at Christmas he refused my Christmas gift, saying I spent too much on him.

On another occasion he called me another girls name when he was saying goodbye. *REALLY A BAD SIGN.* Finally, the clincher on Valentine's Day. I had spent weeks putting together a basket of all the stuff I knew he would like. I was pretty excited to give it to him. When I did give it to him he said I really can't take this from you because I can't have a girlfriend, I'm graduating this year and I can't be in a relationship. *EXCUSE ME?* My thoughts were: thanks-a-f***ing-lot! *HAPPY V-DAY.* I ended up sharing the basket with my other floor mates.

My girlfriends still call him the Toad because he certainly was not my Prince Charming! —THE SLIME THAT MEN DO

Let's Swing Slime Styles
—Anon.

My story begins…

One Valentine's Day, my boyfriend of five months asked me to dress up real sexy. Earlier that day, he got me a spa package, with the full works, manicure, pedicure, wax, hair and make-up done. This was the first time he'd ever done this and he was really excited about what he had planned. I dressed very special that night. Being 22-years-old at the time, it was easy to dress sexy. With my tight black pencil skirt, stilettos and low cut blouse I was ready to go. *I'D SAY (GROWL NOISE)* He picked me up at 10:00 P.M. (hmm too late for dinner) and we slowed down to what seemed to be a bunch of warehouses. I smiled and gave him the benefit of the doubt. Tucked away in the corner was a bar and as we entered the door my heart fell. It was a swinger's party and not only that, an O-L-D-E-R swinger's party. *NICE SURPRISE!!*
—THE SLIME THAT MEN DO

Sad, Slimey and Well, Just Sad
—Christine (No longer heartbroken)

I was with my boyfriend for four years. We met in college, dated for a year then moved in and lived together for three years. I loved him with all my heart he was an amazing man.

It was Valentines Day of 2004 and he had given me a "Promise Ring." He sat me down and promised that he wanted to spend the rest of his life with me and that I meant everything to him. It was the sweetest thing I'd ever experienced. I was on Cloud Nine.

A week later, my boyfriend had said he thought I should go visit my parents, I hadn't seen them in a really long time. I thought oh wow, he is just so perfect. So he drove me home and I spent a week at my parent's house. My boyfriend had called me everyday and said "I love you and miss you so much" and "I can't wait for you to come home." *WHY DO I GET THE FEELING SOMETHING BAD IS ABOUT TO HAPPEN?*

It was a week later when I had my best friend come and pick me up from my parents' house and take me back to our place. My best friend and I walked into my house and it was empty. I'm talking nothing left in the house besides my clothes and my bed. HE MOVED OUT! *(HEAD SHAKING DOUBLE-TAKE!!)*

I was devastated. I tried to call his parents but my phone number had been blocked. I called his cell phone and the number had been disconnected. I went over to his parent's house, knocked on the door as his car was in the driveway. My boyfriend came outside and I was like "what's going on?" and all he said was "I'm not happy and I think we should break up" I didn't have anything to say, I was just in a state of shock.

The next day it hit me hard. I cried for three weeks straight. I lost 45 lbs from not eating. I refused to leave my house I was devastated and heart broken.

I hadn't heard from him and couldn't get a hold of him. It was really over.

Three months later my friends took me to the bar to get me out of the house. My ex-boyfriend just so happened to be there. So of course I went up to him to say hi. To my shock this girl was hanging off him and I kind of gave him a weird look and he said "this is my girlfriend." My mouth dropped open; it had only been three months since he broke up with me. I didn't say anything. I just turned and walked away. I now was not only heart broken but felt horrific and awful.

I am now doing fine and standing on my own two feet. Whatever hurts you can only make you stronger. But I tell ya I think that was pretty slimey of him.

—THE SLIME THAT GUYS WHO BREAK YOUR HEART DO

Another "Worst" Valentine's Story Ever!!!
—Anon.

I was dating this guy and we were planning to spend Valentines Day by having a nice quiet dinner. *OKAY.*

The evening started off badly when he refused to pick me up because he said we were going to be going in the other direction and there was no point in him driving out of his way to my place and then back. So I had to drive to his place. When I got there he told me that before we went for dinner we had to pick up his brother's friend and drop them off at a local bar. *OOOO HOW ROMANTIC...*

I was a little upset but I went along with it. When his brother got in the car he sat on some flowers in the back seat and passed them to me saying "oh sorry I sat on them, I guess they are for you" *NO THEY WERE FOR YOU.*

After picking up his brother's friend we stopped at the bar, where my boyfriend decided we should pop in for a few drinks. So here we were sitting at the bar (not even at a table or booth, no, at the bar) and we order our first round. Then ten minutes later the boys order round two. At this point the brother decided to order food. So the boys all ordered food (including my boyfriend—who never even asked if I wanted anything) By round three the boys were fully involved with whatever was on the TV and I have fallen into a conversation with the guy next to me at the bar. *I'M SORRY IS THIS STILL VALENTINE'S DAY NIGHT? OKAY I JUST RE-READ AND I REALIZE IT IS... WOW THIS IS GOING GREAT!*

At some point my boyfriend decided that he didn't like this guy talking to me. So he got off his stool and decided to pick a fight. He pulled the guy off his barstool and made the first swing (which missed). The guy defended himself and swung back which landed squarely on my boyfriend's temple. He was out cold. *NICE.* So then his brother and friend decided to get the guy back. Needless to say they started a bar fight and got kicked out. Leaving ME with the bill! *OF COURSE THEY DID...*

The bar manager called the cops and took the car's license plate number (the cops later called at the boyfriend's parents place looking for him). When I got outside the guys were waiting at the car. My boyfriend was just coming-to. He was very "out-of-it," he didn't know who or where he was which scared me. The brother and friend wanted to be dropped off at another bar. So I dropped them off and took the boyfriend to the hospital fearing that he had a concussion. When we got to the hospital he could barely walk and by the time we got inside he was delusional. He was immediately admitted with head injuries and they began all sorts of tests. I stayed in the waiting room for nearly 6 hours before I could see him and then after an hour with him the doctors decided to keep him overnight.

I was going to go home but first I had to go to his parents' place and explain to them why there son was in the hospital and why the cops had called. They were not impressed because they were supposed to be leaving on a holiday the following day. And you would think that the story ends. *I'M EXHAUSTED*

NO. The next morning the boyfriend was scheduled to be transferred by ambulance to another hospital for a CAT scan and I was going to meet him at the other hospital in case he was released from there. But before he was transferred he left the hospital against medical advice. I had his car and cell phone so he walked to a payphone and called a cab. I spent two hours at the hospital looking for him before a nurse found out why he had never arrived. So that evening I went over to his house to make sure he was okay and he gave me crap because I had brought him to a hospital, taken his car back home instead of waiting all night, and because he left his cell in the car, it was also my fault that he had to use a payphone. *WOW, THIS GUY IS SUCH A DICK ON SO MANY LEVELS...*

I think I had the worst Valentines ever because: *LET'S REVIEW IN CASE THOSE OF YOU AT HOME HAVE GOTTEN LOST...*

1. Boyfriend refused to pick me up—I was too far "out-of-the-way"
2. Had to play the taxi role for brother and friend
3. Boyfriend brother gave me my flowers after sitting on them
4. Boyfriend ate at the BAR and we never made it to a restaurant so I didn't even get a dinner
5. Boyfriend ignored me all night
6. Boyfriend picked a fight
7. Boyfriend lost the fight, got knocked out cold and got kicked out of the bar
8. Boyfriend, brother and friend all LEFT ME WITH THE BILL!!!
9. Boyfriend was admitted to hospital with serious concussion, and head trauma
10. I spent more than six hours in the hospital
11. I had to go explain to his parents what had happened and why the cops called
12. Boyfriend left AMA (and didn't tell me)
13. I spent over two hours looking for boyfriend at hospital
14. Boyfriend blamed me for the evening!?

Needless to say I am not with this guy anymore. *NO! I WOULD HAVE GUESSED YOU AND SLIMEO WOULD HAVE LIVED HAPPILY EVER AFTER!!!*
—THE SLIME THAT (*SEE 1 THROUGH 14 ABOVE*) DO!!!

Guys Get Slimed Too.
—Zane Qureshi

Last Valentines, my girlfriend and I had a romantic night planned—dinner for two in front of a live jazz band, dancing, a nice walk along the lakeshore. *NICE TOUCH.* It seemed pretty sweet at the time.

So Valentine's Day nears and my girlfriend ends our relationship. She leaves me a message saying how things aren't working out. *CHICKY BREAKS UP ON THIS DUDES MACHINE...COLD.* I however, do not check my messages and I am still planning this romantic evening. *YOU JUST KNOW THIS IS NOT GOING TO END WELL.*

So the big V day arrives and instead of calling her to tell her I'm coming I thought I'd surprise her, you know play the sweet guy role, and come early with flowers. I still hadn't heard the message and she opens the door with one of her friends of the opposite sex. Completely flustered, I felt the only thing to do was to leave. But just my luck, I locked my keys in my car. Ironically, the guy she was with is a tow-truck driver and he unlocked the door. *HANDY.* Quite humiliating. *THAT TOO...* I left the feeling 'stupid.' I learned my lesson now I keep my cell phone with me at all times.   —THE SLIME THAT WOMEN DO

More Valentine's Horror Stories
—Sandy Watson

This Valentine's Day horror story happened quite a few years ago, but it was so incredibly bad that it has stuck in my mind for all this time. *OKAY, LET'S GO BACK IN TIME TO THE SCENE OF THE SLIME...*

I decided to make my significant other (at the time) a very romantic dinner. I chose barbecued steak, baked potatoes, sauteed mushrooms, fresh vegetables, caesar salad and a homemade cherry cheesecake. *(STOMACH NOISES—GURGLE... GURGLE... ETC.)*

I began by turning on the stove but I had forgotten to take off the metal element cover. I had to use a fork to flip it off because it was already burning hot. When I flipped it, it fell on the floor and burnt the linoleum. Okay, I got past that problem and pushed on. When I started up the barbecue, I had a wonderful flame going but unfortunately the flames were coming from under the barbecue—all around the tank and the base of the barbecue. *THAT'S NOT GOOD.* I had to use a fire extinguisher to put it out. Luckily my neighbor had a barbecue that I could use and managed to cook the steaks anyway! I am no quitter! I finally get the dinner made (without burning down the whole house) and I set the table, pour the wine, and light the candles, yes that is right, I lit the candles! When I went back into the kitchen to put the final touches on the meal, one of the candles fell over and lit the table cloth on fire. *JIM CAREY CAN PLAY YOU IN THE MOVIE.* I managed to put that out with very little damage.

My other half came home and dinner actually turned out quite well. We both ate it with no other major disasters. So, here is the best part of my evening—right after desert, he decided that he was going to watch a hockey game with a buddy. *ON VALENTINE'S DAY NIGHT? ARE YOU KIDDING?* No, it was not a NHL game or anything, just a local house league team. So in spite of all the trauma, I managed to make a very good meal, not go insane and not have to call the fire department and I all I got in return was a sink full of dishes and an evening all by myself...*COURTESY OF...*   —THE SLIME THAT MEN DO

A Redneck Valentine's Day, Yeehaw
—Bree Walsh

I think I'm gonna take the cake with this one. I just moved to Toronto from North Carolina. I married a Canadian, thankfully, who rescued me from having to endure yet another redneck Valentine's Day.

A few years ago, long before I met my Canadian husband of course, I was dating Timmy. Even the name fits! It was an unusually warm February so I was thinking a picnic by the lake, a nice walk to the ice cream shop, etc, etc. Timmy talked up the day for weeks. He kept saying that he was going to sweep me off my feet, that I just better be ready to be romanced. I was darn well gettin' excited! *I'M DURN WELL GETTING EXCITED TOO!*

The day arrived. Around lunchtime, Timmy came over with a box wrapped with a big red bow. The box was cool to the touch, so I was thinkin' chocolates? When the bow came off, I realized the box was stamped by the local bait shop, which I just knew had to be because it was the only box Timmy could find. Nope! It was a box of fresh, squirmy, live worms! *NO CHOCOLATES?* He smiled, threw out his arms like it was the big finale, and yelled that he was "takin' me fishin'!" I was wondering why he'd shown up for our romantic dinner in a camouflage hat and matching pants. I changed out of my stiletto heels and into some rubber boots and went with Timmy, hoping things would get better. He had a 12 pack waitin' in the cooler in the truck and poles in the back. *12 PACKS CAN BE ROMANTIC?*

This was no romantic row boat on the lake either. Timmy got drunk and fell asleep with his pole between his legs. He woke up only for a second to tell me to "wake him up if he got a bite." Needless to say that was the last Valentine Day for me and Timmy!

—THE SLIME THAT JETHRO'S DO

Stop Yelling At The Screen!
—Heather

The one and only time I went on a first date on Valentine's Day the guy took me to a movie, not even for a mushy girlie movie, it was some Arnold or Sylvester thing. Well, everything was going great until the guy I was with stood up in the middle of the movie and start yelling at the screen, not just "don't go in there" type of things, it was more like "what have I been telling you, she's the enemy. It might help if you listen to me!!!" *DID THE DUDE THINK THE MOVIE COULD HEAR HIM? WAS THIS HIS FIRST TIME IN A THEATRE?* I was so freaked out!!

Everyone started yelling at him to shut up and sit down, I was so embarrassed I didn't even know what to say, but by the tone of his voice and the look on his face I was certain that it was no joke!! *OH THIS JUST SOUNDS LIKE TONS OF FUN!!* I told him that I had to go to the bathroom and I never came back, I was too embarrassed!! *NO KIDDING*

Now three years later I'm moving in with a wonderful man who would never even think to do something like that! *MOST MEN WOULDN'T DO THE SLIME THAT GUYS THAT YELL AT THE SCREEN IN MOVIES WOULD DO*

#17

Hey, Where'd Jim Go?
—Samantha

I had been dating a particular guy for about three months (let's call him Jim) *OKAY.*

On Valentine's Day, Jim told me to be ready at 6:30 and he would be by to pick me up. Excited to see what surprises awaited me, I was ready to go by 6. My doorbell rang, and there he was....with his best friend. *SURPRISE!* Apparently, Jim's car had broken down and he was supposed to drop his friend off at his girlfriend's house. Jim figured I could drive us and his friend.

After dropping off his friend, we went to Don Valentino's, a really nice (and expensive) place in Brampton. Jim told me to order anything I wanted... so I did. And so did he... appetizers, drinks, dinner, dessert. The evening was wonderful. The food was spectacular and I had practically forgotten about the night's earlier stumbles. Until the bill came. *UH OH.* Jim looked over the bill, cringed, and excused himself to the bathroom. Somehow, he managed to sneak out the front door, leaving me with the bill. *NO WAY.* And the embarrassment of explaining that my date had slipped out on me. *HE DID A DINE-AND-DASH ON VALENTINES DAY?* I left, a little red faced and a little light in the wallet. Needless to say, Jim received many calls over the next few days but did not return any of them. The relationship was over, but I had hoped to at least give him a piece of my mind. I never did seem Jim again. Probably better that way. *FOR YOU AND FOR JIM.*

Thankfully, I have found a wonderful man that never slips out on the bill. However, I figured it couldn't be a bad thing to let women know that there are some Jim's out there, and to watch out for them! They could run to the bathroom at any time! *EVEN IF THEY DON'T HAVE TO PEE… THE SLIME THAT MEN WHO DECIDE THAT THE BILL IS TOO MUCH AND NOW MIGHT BE A GOOD TIME TO BREAK UP AND LEAVE WITHOUT PAYING THE BILL DO.*

A Very Strange Tale of Romance That Actually Ends Well
—Jorgina Ribau

I went to a Valentine's Day dance and met a guy there. Afterward a bunch of us went to the local McDonald's. I sat with my friends and he sat with his and through the entire time at the restaurant he kept bunching up paper napkins and throwing them at me. *THAT'S WHAT BOYS DO WHEN THEY LIKE A GIRL… WAS HE 12??* A friend of mine that I was with got really upset when one hit her and decided it was time for us to leave. We all got up to leave and so did he. We got in the car and he kept asking me for my phone number. *WELL OF COURSE, AFTER ALL HE HAD THROWN WADED UP PAPER NAPKINS AT YOU!!* I told him that I didn't want to give it to him but he wouldn't take no for an answer. He threw himself in front of the car and laid down on the ground and said he wouldn't get up until he got my phone number. *OKAY KIND OF COOL.* His friends were all watching and couldn't stop laughing. Frustrated that we couldn't go anywhere, one of my friends rolled down the window and shouted out my phone number to him. He then shouted out as we drove off that he would give me a call on Valentine's Day.

Well as weird as it sounds, I waited on Valentines Day for his phone call. *WHY NOT, HE YELLED FROM A MACDONALD'S PARKING LOT THAT HE WOULD CALL.* I waited all night near the phone and no phone call. The following week he called me and I told him that I waited all night on Valentines day for his phone call and he thought it was funny. *SO OF COURSE YOU TOLD HIM OFF AND NEVER SAW HIM AGAIN RIGHT???* To make a long story short, we have been together for 16 years and married for almost 14 years and have three boys together. *OR THAT.*

Hopefully none of them will take after their father in the romance department. *WHY NOT, IT WORKED FOR HIM…THE SLIME THAT GUYS THAT YOU TURN OUT MARRYING DO*

Curling, Computers and Slime!
—Jenifer Gault

Mike and I were going out for over a year at the time and were both going to school. I lived at home and commuted while he lived in res and we both had jobs. *OKAY, AS ALWAYS, SOUND FINE SO FAR… (CUE: OMINOUS MUSIC DUN DUN DUHHHHHHHHH)* Anyway, in preparation for Valentine's day I bought some new lingerie, I got my hair done, and I bought him a beautiful lighter with his name engraved on it. I spent a lot of time shopping for it btw. *LIGHTERS ARE NICE, NOT AS SEXY AS LINGERIE BUT…*

Valentine's Day came, and I was super excited. I couldn't wait to see Mike! After his class, I went to his room to give him his gift. He said "thanks!" then went back to his Olympic Curling. *SQUEEZE ME, DID YOU SAY CURLING, AS IN ROCKS AND BROOMS?* Yes, that's right CURLING!

I said "why don't we do something"… his response? He whined "but Jennnnn… it's OLYMPIC curling" (I'd just like to point out that he NEVER watched any sports on TV… NONE! And this was the only Olympic event he watched that year… the guy was a computer geek!) *WELL IT WAS OLYMPIC CURLING, GEEZ.*

So there I sat, looking great with sexies on under my clothes, riding up my Bum, watching curling. I went and picked up Chinese for a romantic dinner after Curling was done. Nope! He switched it to some computer show. And he didn't even offer to pay for the food since he didn't get me a gift or even a card. *AND THIS SOMEHOW DIDN'T MEET YOUR VALENTINES DAY EXPECTATIONS??*

The next morning I got up early, drove home and cried for hours. There was never an apology... just the complaint that I had spelled "Michael" wrong on his lighter. *YOUR KIDDING RIGHT?* The next week-end I drove him and his buddies to a computers flea market and he bought me a modem as a "belated Valentine's gift" for $15. It didn't end up working. What a find!

—The Slime That Computer Geeks Who Like Curling Do

Surprise! We've Both Bee Slimed
—Chris Corcoran (a dude)

Last year for Valentines Day I decided to surprise my girlfriend with a Jacuzzi suite for the night. So I booked the suite and got everything we would need: dinner, candles and alcohol—the works. I was told over the phone that I could do an early check-in (2:00 P.M.) instead of the normal 4 P.M. check-in. However when I got there at 2:00, I was told that they weren't allowing early check ins today and to come back later. *OKAY.* I was temporarily baffled, but I left and returned at 4 PM when I was given the key to my Jacuzzi suite. When I opened the door and looked around I noticed there was a single rose on top of the TV, two champagne glasses on the table, and three candles lining the Jacuzzi bathtub. This was unexpected and helpful. *SETTING A NICE MOOD!* While we were "relaxing" *YOU MEAN "DOIN IT?"* there was a knock at the door, then another. I got up and someone was trying to open the door! If I hadn't used the chain they would have seen me shocked and naked in all my glory! I told them to hold on and I put on some clothes and looked out the peep hole. *OH, YOU MEAN IN THE DOOR. OH THAT MAKES SENSE.*

When I looked out of peep hole I saw a woman with a bag of groceries and her husband as well as the lady from the front desk waiting not so patiently. When I finally opened the door the woman stated that this was their room! It turns out that those champagne glasses were hers. The rose atop the TV, hers. The three candles that lined the Jacuzzi, yep, those were hers too! So we had to allow these people to come in and collect their belongings. Some other employee at the front desk made the mistake of giving this couple their keys earlier in the day, they deposited a few belongings and left to buy food. This is how my Valentines Day 2004 was a complete and total disaster.

—The Slime That Uh Well Someone Got Slimed By Somebody!

Valentine Slime From Hell
—Nancy Slawski

Several years ago, a very insistent and persistent co-worker nagged me so much that I gave in and went out on a blind date, my very first and only blind date, on Valentine's Day. Yes, in retrospect I can see that I must have been temporarily insane to ever agree to such a thing. *NO KIDDING.*

The guy, she said, was a good friend of her husband (note: I had yet to meet her husband so I wasn't as leery as I should have been). The description that my co-worker gave me of the guy was of someone I probably had nothing in common with on any level, but for some reason, I blame it on a cold and dreary February, I agreed. *THESE THINGS HAPPEN, HOW BAD COULD IT BE???*

The big day rolls around and I showed up at my co-workers house, where we were meeting before dinner. Once I met her husband, I know that this was a bad idea, because after one look at him (oily bohunk variety) *BOHUNK? THAT DOESN'T SOUND LIKE A GOOD THING* and one very short conversation I knew that his friends weren't exactly 'ideal' date material. So, there I am and there we are, waiting for the friend to show up, one hour, two hours, no show. The husband calls the guy, and guess what—he completely blew off the date. *OHH THAT BAD... WOW.*

So there I am dumped by guy I didn't even want to date to begin with, on Valentine's Day. *THAT'S JUST PLAIN MEAN.*

But wait, the story doesn't end there. After discovering that I'd been dumped, I decided it was best that I just head home but the couple would not hear of it, and insisted I join them for dinner. I declined, but the co-worker made such a big deal about it, and insisted I'd love the restaurant, and that it would be her treat—so very reluctantly, I allowed myself to become the third wheel on a Valentine's date. *THIS IS GETTING WORSE BY THE MINUTE.* We get to the restaurant, it's in a shady area of the city, one that I'm sure no cabs would come to if I decided I wanted to leave. Anyway, we sit down, I order the seafood marinara and I listen to this couple argue throughout the entire meal. Finally, the meal is done, I end up paying for my crappy meal, and my evening from hell looks like it's almost over, or so it seems. I got home, went to bed, and after a few hours I find myself sprinting to the bathroom, where I spent the reminder of February 14th and part of February 15th—I had food poisoning. *HAPPY VALENTINES DAY!!! THE SLIME THAT COUPLES WHO SET YOU UP ON A BLIND DATE WITH A DUDE WHO DOESN'T EVEN SHOW AND THEN DRAG YOU TO A PLACE WHERE THE FOOD MAKES YOU SICK... DO.*

#22

Eva's Personal Valentine Nightmare Slime
—Eva Golen

A few years ago a new love had to go away on a business trip to Florida for a whole week around Valentine's Day and asked if I would like to join him. He said that he was going to drive down since he was more relaxed driving his fully loaded Navigator than flying. He said that he would love my company on the drive down and that during the day while he was at meetings I could shop and sunbathe but that the nights would be for us—delicious dinners, romantic walks, moonlight swims, not to mention bubble baths and champagne in our hotel! *SOUNDS GREAT.* He made everything sound so romantic and exciting that I jumped at the chance to go with him; after all, we'd had dates, but no real intimacy. *NO YOU KNOW, "RELATIONS"* This would be our first overnight trip together and right around Valentine's Day too!! I said that I would LOVE to go with him. Before the trip, I had my hair done, got a manicure, pedicure and waxed all the right parts of my body. I shopped for comfortable, yet sexy car clothes, soft and silky lingerie, not to mention seven days' worth of different matching bras and panties. *THAT'S HOW I ROLL.*

We left on a bright sunny day and started driving south. We made it as far as Cincinnati the first night and found a nice hotel to stay in for the night. He was full of surprises. After dinner, he ran a bubble bath for me and when I emerged from my leisurely soak, I found that he had brought candles and they were lit and softly glowing all over the room. He handed me a glass of wine and left me for a short while so that he could shower. *IT'S ALMOST TOO PERFECT.* We made love that night in a candlelit room with the hum of the Interstate in the distance. The night was perfect. I wouldn't have changed a thing. He was great kisser and a kind, considerate and generous lover. *MUCH LIKE MYSELF !* I couldn't believe that I would be lucky enough to have a whole week of this kind of bliss and pampering! What a great Valentine's it was going to be!! *NO KIDDING.*

The next morning was Valentine's Day. When we woke up he said that he wasn't feeling good and that he decided to cancel the trip and turn around and go back home. *WHAT THE???* I was shocked! He didn't appear sick. He wasn't doubled over in pain, or throwing up or anything. He said he didn't have a headache, migraine, fever, backache or anything. He wasn't even sniffling for Pete's sake. I suggested a trip to a drugstore but he said no, he just wanted to go home. I had no idea what was going on. *VERY WEIRD.* We drove home our second day pretty much in silence, except for me asking him how he was feeling. He dropped me off at home and that was it. I never heard from him again. *????????????*

—THE SLIME THAT EVEN SEEMINGLY PERFECT MEN DO

Not Slimey As Much As Just Some Bad Valentines Luck
—Diane D.

Three years ago my boyfriend, now fiancé, and I decided to go to a Valentine's Day formal put on by my department at University. *FORMALS ARE FUN… WHAT ARE FORMALS?* We decided to go all out; he rented a tux, I pulled out a formal gown and had my hair done. Needless to say, we spent a bit of money on this plan. Well, we arrived at the hotel where the formal was to take place, dressed to the nines, and we can't see the party listed anywhere on the hotel directory. So, we ask the receptionist. She's never heard of this formal. I began to wonder if I'd read my tickets incorrectly, but they're right in my hand and this is the place, time, and date. The receptionist goes to look into it and returns looking very apologetic and replies that the formal has been cancelled. *CANCELLED FORMALS ARE NO FUN!* Apparently I hadn't received the e-mail stating this. Well, fine, the night won't be a total waste, since we're all dressed up, why not go out for a fancy dinner instead? Do you know how hard it is to get dinner reservations at 7 P.M. on Valentines Day? *VERY HARD?* We call a hotel and book a room, right after finally finding a nice restaurant. Everything seems to be going swell. We decided to check on the hotel before we eat, just to be sure of which one it was (this is in Niagara Falls, and there are three hotels from the same chain). The hotel receptionist assures us that there is no booking under my name, and that the confirmation number we gave him was not one that they use. Well, whatever, we've got dinner reservations and there's still one more hotel in the city, so off we go. *SOUNDS LIKE EVERYTHING WILL HAVE TO BE FINE NOW, WON'T IT?*

We arrive at the restaurant and are seated (so far, so good) and we wait for our waitress… and we wait… and a waitress approaches… and goes to the table next to us… and we wait… and the couple next to us have finished their meal… and we wait. My boyfriend gets up and speaks with the hostess, and not long afterward a flustered waitress appears claiming that she didn't know we were there. Finally, we eat.

The waitress brings a shot of Sambuca to apologize for being late to our table, and as it turns out my boyfriend hates Sambuca. **OH NO.** So, we're ready to turn in at this point. My boyfriend runs across the street to the other hotel to check on our reservation, and he returns with the same news as the last hotel. I'm worried now because I had given out my credit card number what now seems to be an imaginary hotel. We're told that there's one more hotel in the city. We go there and they check, and no, there's no reservation for me. But, the receptionist takes pity on the poor young couple all dressed up with nowhere to go, and she finds out which hotel I had so unwittingly given my credit card information to. As it turns out, it was in another city, but it wasn't too far away so off we go again. (I'm glad gas was cheaper then.)

Finally, we get to the hotel and we're bringing our bags inside. Nothing could POSSIBLY go wrong now. Oh, wait. I can still feel it. I lost my balance holding open the door, took a step back, my body lurches forward for balance and *rip*. Oh yes, I had just torn my expensive formal gown. **THAT HAPPENED TO ME ONCE!** Well, I'm sorry but I had had enough at that point and was forced to cry. **ME TOO.** So much for romance. We haven't celebrated Valentines Day since. In fact, we make a point of watching bad action films and eating greasy, spicy pizza on Feb 14th.

—THE UH... SLIME THAT UH... HAPPENS TO
COUPLES ON VALENTINE'S DAY UH DO?

You're So Slime
—Kerin Donahue

Please find attached my Valentine's Day Nightmare Date story. I am no longer allowed to play the 'who had the worst date ever' game with my friends because I always win.

Last year on Valentine's Day I found myself single and fancy-free. I wasn't desperate, just a little at loose ends on what to do on the most pressure-filled day of the year for single people. So I decided to accept a date through one of those on-line dating sites. Okay, so maybe 'desperate' is a fair assessment. **NO ONE'S JUDGING.** I took him to my favourite 'first date' place—a nice bistro and pool bar. He showed up, tried to cop a feel in the first five minutes and then downed four beers and four shots in forty minutes. **YOU'RE MAKING THAT UP.**

At first glance I thought I had done fairly well—the guy was reasonably good-looking, with acceptable hygiene levels. The second he opened his mouth, however, I realized I had made a horrible, horrible mistake: if Randy 'Macho Man' Savage and The "Duff" Man from the *Simpsons* had had a love child, he was standing right in front of me. **I DIDN'T EVEN KNOW THEY WERE DATING!**

He was a 'close talker'; someone who has to stand no less than 6 inches in front of your nose. He also shouted absolutely everything and, if he had just taken a swig of his beer, some of that liquid would invariably land on my face. **EWWWWW!** His truly memorable trade-mark was that he kept repeating the same phrase at completely random intervals: "you're so hot! You're so ultimate! Ohhhh yeah!" **YOUR SO KIDDING RIGHT?** He repeated this over and over and over again, in a hearty bellow that made the fixtures in the bar rattle.

He became so intoxicated he could barely stand. At one point, during a coughing fit, I thought he was going to throw up on the bar. While playing a game of pool, I looked down to see his hand on my purse. At first I thought he was trying to swipe my wallet. In fact, he was actually caressing it, as he had mistaken my leather shoulder bag for my butt. **THAT'S JUST FUNNY.**

Halfway through our miserable game he went to visit the facilities. While enjoying the break, the bartender came up to me and asked me to leave. I was embarrassed; I thought that he was kicking us out because my psychotic date was disturbing the other patrons. He corrected me, "No, the rest of the staff and I have been watching. We think *you* should leave. As in, sneak out. Don't worry about the bill; we'll take care of it. Just get out while you can. Please, we're begging you." **NO WAY!** I looked toward the bar and saw a collection of bar-tenders and wait staff sadly shaking their heads at me and making 'shoo-ing' motions towards the exit. **THIS IS SO GREAT.**

Well, I did not take their advice. I was determined to be polite and finish the date with my head held high. Fifty-seven 'you're so hot', later, we finally left. He followed me to my car, despite several hints from me that this was not necessary. When we got there, I said good night and good-bye. He looked at me, disbelieving, and said, "What? We're not going back to your place for a hot-hot romp between the sheets?" I firmly informed him that this was not the case. *YOU-HAVE-JUST-GOT-TO-BE-MAKING-THIS-UP!!* He was astonished. "But it's Valentine's Day! Everyone knows that on Valentine's Day chicks get really horny and have to have sex if they don't have a boyfriend or husband. I figured you were a sure thing! What are you a lesbian or something?" People, if any of you had a quiet moment last Valentine's day and you heard a loud "WHAT????" reverberating across the cosmos… yeah. That was me. I went home. Expeditiously. When I arrived, I had a new e-mail waiting for me, from him that consisted of one word which I cannot repeat. *I'LL BET HE MISSPELLED IT…*

—The Slime That Drunken Nitwits Do

The Twisted Tale of Complicated Slime
—Mike Di Savino

First I'll have to introduce the people involved in the story:
- Mike (myself)
- Sandy (now my wife)
- Chrissy (my ex-girlfriend)
- Richard (Sandy's ex-boyfriend)
- Bret (Sandy's way at getting back at me)

HI EVERYBODY I'M HOWARD.

So, let's start at the beginning. I dated Chrissy for almost seven years, splitting up about three times. Sandy dated Richard for four-plus years, also splitting up a few times. *OKAY* I met Sandy working at McDonald's about five years ago. We were both happily dating our significant others at the time. Then things started getting shaky for both of us in our relationships. So when we had decided to date other people, we started to date each other. *I'M ALREADY LOST.* Anyway ... we dated each other and our ex's for about a year. Then I finally got back together with Chrissy on New Year's Eve. Sandy didn't go back to Richard just yet, she decided to date other people because she knew that I still cared for her and it would drive me nuts. *SURE. WHICH ONE IS MIKE AGAIN?*

So, on Valentine's Day I have a big fight with Chrissy the night before and she dumped me on the phone. This couldn't have been better news for me. I immediately hung up and called Sandy (my one true love) and told her the news. Unfortunately she had already made plans with her pot-head fling Bret. *WHO THE HELL IS BRET?* So I begged her to let me pick her up after her date because this loser didn't have a car. So she let me. Earlier on during that day Sandy was with Richard at Yorkdale buying Valentine's gifts but not for him, for Bret and me. *WAIT A SECOND, YOU'RE DATING BRET?* Did I mention that it was also Richard's birthday on Feb. 14th? *YOU MIGHT HAVE BUT I WAS STILL TRYING TO FIGURE OUT HOW TO GET BRET OFF THE WEED!* Sucks to be him. Anyway, he catches her buying gifts for the other two men in her life and kind of freaks out. They part ways and Sandy goes to Bret's apartment and exchanges gifts. I meet with Chrissy to clear things up. *OH I'M SURE THINGS WERE CRYSTAL CLEAR BY THIS POINT.* I wanted to make sure that she knew we were breaking up. She denied dumping me but I didn't want to hear it. I gave her a card but just signed the back of it. I usually write something in it. I also told her that I had bought her Mamma Mia tickets for later on that month but wasn't going to bring her. So I went to pick-up Sandy, gave her the perfect Valentine's Day gift and told her that I was done with Chrissy and that I would be taking her to Mamma Mia instead of Chrissy. From that day on Sandy and I have been happily together and now married for more than one year and expecting our first child. *WHAT HAPPENED TO RICHARD, CHRISSY AND BRET... TUNE IN NEXT TIME FOR THE SLIME THAT... OH FORGET IT LET'S JUST GIVE BRET A CALL AND WATCH A FUNNY MOVIE!!!*

Real "Slime" With A Happy Ending!!!

Dave and Trudy Hepburn spent their Valentine's Day digging through garbage to find a diamond pendant!!

While away on vacation, Trudy kept her very sentimental heart shaped pendant in a fanny pack, wrapped in a piece of tissue, along with her ID and other valuables to protect it from being lost or stolen. When they returned from vacation, Dave emptied the fanny pack of valuable items on the kitchen counter. On Valentine's Day, Trudy asked Dave for the fanny pack so that she could wear the pendant. When Dave told his wife that he had emptied all items on the counter, Trudy realized she had thrown the tissue and pendant into the garbage!

Dave had taken the garbage bags to the curb that very morning!! When they discovered that the garbage had already been picked up that day, they called Halton Regional Landfill. Yes, their garbage truck had been there, had emptied the garbage, and a bulldozer was already crushing it!! With the assistance of two women and two men from the site, they looked through the garbage that had come off the garbage truck. Dave distinctly remembered that the garbage bag they were looking for was light green and contained four white kitchen-catchers.

After some time working in the rain and cold, the landfill crew realized that this was the wrong pile, and that the garbage truck from Dave and Trudy's neighborhood had dumped somewhere else, along with eight other trucks. After picking the most likely pile, the search begins again! Finding mail that was addressed to a neighbor brings hope that this is the right pile! When Dave finds a light green bag, containing four kitchen catchers, and an odd sock that he had thrown out the week before, he realizes that this is his garbage!! Indeed, they find a piece of tissue paper, with the diamond pendant tucked inside!!! The people at the Halton Region Landfill were not only very helpful, but they also ran the story of the lost pendant in their newsletter!! How do you top this for next Valentine's Day Dave ??? *SOMETIMES THINGS GET SLIMEY FOR MEN EVEN WHEN THEY'RE NOT TRYING.*

Have your own **STUPID CUPID** story?

E-mail your story to **slime@humblehoward.com** and it could be included in our next book, *The Slime That Men Do 2!*

Here, make some notes, it could be therapeutic:

_____

_____

_____

_____

_____

_____

_____

_____

_____

_____

_____

_____

_____

_____

_____

_____

_____

_____